The Red Thread of Pilates:
The Mat©

STUDY GUIDE

TOOLS TO FACILITATE A DEEPER UNDERSTANDING AND
LOGICAL PROGRESSION OF STUDY THROUGH THE
PILATES MAT REPERTOIRE AS PRESENTED IN
"THE RED THREAD OF PILATES"©

Tracy Maurstad

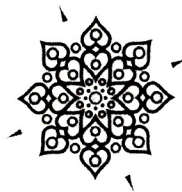

zest and pleasure
publications

DEDICATION

To the one and only Kathryn Ross-Nash, for giving us all
a peek into your marvelous Pilates brain.
Thank you for so generously sharing your incredible wealth of knowledge.

TABLE OF CONTENTS

DISCLAIMER

THIS STUDY GUIDE is intended to be used as a companion reference to
Kathryn Ross-Nash's book "The Red Thread of Pilates -
The Integrated System and Variations of Pilates: The Mat"©.

Kathi's book is a comprehensive resource for the Pilates Mat repertoire.
The purpose of this guide is to facilitate a logical progression of study through Kathi's book.
It is not intended to be used as a separate resource.

1. ABOUT "THE RED THREAD OF PILATES: THE MAT" ©

CONGRATULATIONS. YOU INVESTED in the "Red Thread of Pilates: The Mat©" by Kathryn Ross-Nash. You hold a comprehensive Mat workshop from one of the great teachers and practitioners of The Pilates Method in your hands. That's how I think of it anyway - like an incredible Mat workshop with Kathi that would take many days, if not weeks, to complete, along with the world's greatest notes. But OMG it's huge. It's monstrous! Threads? Add Next numbers? Variations, variations and more variations. The Hundred takes 5 pages. Seriously? How am I supposed to get my head around all this information?!

Kathi's approach is very logical, but for many teachers it's a new way of seeing the repertoire. So if you find it all a bit overwhelming, or if the overall structure of the book isn't crystal clear, you are not alone. Because it can be so new and there's so much information to assimilate it can be useful to have a sort of Cliffs Notes version; so here we go…

Joseph Pilates gave us the ultimate order in which the mat exercises are performed in his book "Return to Life", but I dare say it's not the order you'd teach them to a new student. I mean, The Roll Over is the third exercise. I don't think so. When you're teaching the mat repertoire to a new student, the third mat exercise you teach them is not The Roll Over. You skip right over The Roll Over and teach them something more basic, maybe a version of the Single Leg Circle. Down the road, once they've built their strength and understanding of how to safely suspend their spine, when you have confidence they won't injure themselves, then you introduce them to The Roll Over. When that time comes, if that time comes, once the Roll Over has been added to their mat workout, then they'll perform the exercise third, after Roll Up (assuming you follow the Classical order). Even if you're a Contemporary teacher and don't teach the original order for the mat work, you still don't introduce new exercises to students in the order they'll ultimately perform them years down their Pilates road. So, no matter your Pilates style, you introduce exercises in a different order than the order in which they'll ultimately be performed. Ok, then, so if the orders are different, then how do you decide which exercise is logical to add next to your/your student's mat workout?

That's what Kathi's done. She's put the entire mat repertoire in an order you'd likely introduce it to a new student. That order is what Kathi calls the "Add Next" number. If you look at the Table of Contents of *The Red Thread©* on page 17-18 the number in parentheses after the exercise name is the "Add Next" number; it also appears after the exercise name at the top of the first page for that exercise. On pages 15 and 16 of this Study Guide you'll find a table of all the exercises in their Add Next order - "Exercises by Order of Introduction ("Add Next")".

On that same table on pages 15 and 16 you'll also see the *thread(s)* for each exercise. There are many ways to categorize the Pilates repertoire. Kathi uses the spine function to segment the repertoire. Each spinal function is a *thread*; what the spine does during an exercise determines what *thread* it belongs to. Basic level exercises usually only belong to one thread, more advanced exercise require multiple movements in the spine so they belong to multiple threads. The threads are Stability (S); Articulation (A); Side Bending (SB); Twisting (T); Extension (E); and Rolling (R) - some Forward (RF), and some in Extension (RE). Each exercise has an Add Next number, its order of introduction. And each exercise has a position within each thread to which it belongs. You'll find the thread sequence number in *The Red Thread©* on the first page for each exercise, in the red box in the upper-left corner. For instance if it says S3, it's the third exercise in the Stability Thread. Starting on page 17 of this Study Guide you'll find separate tables for each *thread* with the exercises in their thread sequence order.

The *threads* provide guidance in building your student's mat workouts. It's highly unlikely you or your student will have the exercises introduced in the exact order listed in Kathi's book. The *Add Next* numbers aren't rules, they're only guidelines. We all have strengths and weaknesses and issues which will impact the order in which exercises get added to our mat workouts, and some students have physical limitations which will eliminate entire threads from their workouts. This is when the "THREAD" order becomes important. If a student does well at a particular thread, they will progress through that *thread* faster than threads they find more challenging. You continue to progress them through what they're able to do, but if an exercise is already a challenge you don't want to progress them deeper down that path to an even more difficult exercise; the beauty of Pilates is that it builds on itself, it is not a disjointed collection of exercises. So, if you get to an exercise they can't adequately perform then you back up and use earlier exercises of that thread (and exercises on other apparatus) to address what needs strengthening, until they're finally ready to continue deeper into that thread.

For an example of how to use the *threads* to help formulate your/your student's mat work, this is from Introduction to the Neck Pull (Add Next #19): "Assisted Teaser Preps prepares the spine for this difficult abdominal exercise and deep stretch." Introduction to the Neck Pull is the seventh exercise in the Articulation thread (A7), the Assisted Teasers are Articulation exercises 3-6 (A3-A6). If Introduction to Neck Pull is too difficult, then you do not add this exercise to the mat workout, you do not progress deeper into the Articulation Thread. You don't build strength with an exercise they *cannot* do, you regress back through the thread to find an exercise they *can* perform. You use those earlier exercises in the *thread,* and exercises on other apparatus, to build what the student needs. Ok, so you're not adding Add Next exercise #19. But the progress through all of the mat exercises doesn't stop, just those in the *Articulation* thread. Add Next exercise #20 is Side Kicks - Up & Down, a Stability and Side Bending exercise (S9 and SB1). The student has good stability so you go ahead and teach them Side Kick – Up & Down, Add Next #20. They are able to adequately perform Side Kick Up & Down so it gets added to their mat routine. Down the road, when the Assisted Teasers and apparatus work have done their job to strengthen the student's ability to articulate, then you go back to Introduction to Neck Pull, Add Next #19 and, if all goes well, continue to progress through the Articulation Thread.

As Kathi states in the opening pages of the book "Every list and all charts are intended to create thought, not hard fast rules. Each exercise has a number, which indicates what exercises to Add Next to create a balanced workout. These numbers are only **suggestions** (emphasis mine) that logically develop the work utilizing the spinal functions and build according to difficulty." So choose thoughtfully which exercise should be added next for you/your student based on the individual's strengths and challenges, using the *threads* as your guide for what exercises to add, or not, to their individual workout. Never strictly adhere to any order of introduction because it happens to have the next *Add Next* number.

Now, what is it with all these variations? Many Pilates teacher trainings these days teach only one variation of an exercise and there's a lot of focus during the training on the particular choreography of that program's version of an exercise. All this focus on the one right way to do an exercise does provide fuel to the Pilates infighting fires…no, THIS is the correct arm position for this exercise! But Kathi makes it clear there is no *one* way to perform most exercises. Almost every exercise has variations designed to address the particular needs of the student. Do they need to open their chest? Stretch their hips? Maybe they round their shoulders or are prone to stretch too far? How do you vary the exercise to suit the student without losing the purpose of the exercise? The variations Kathi presents are for a reason, not just for variety's sake. Kathi has given us tried and true variations that she learned in her many years working closely with Romana Kryzanowska and other first generation Pilates teachers.

On the first page of every exercise page in *The Red Thread©* are the Goal Instructions for that exercise. Think of the Goal Instructions as the Baseline Variation of the exercise ("Baseline Variation" is my term, not Kathi's). Most exercises will also have several Building Variations and Challenge Variations. Building

Variations are used to build the strength required to perform the Baseline Variation (the Goal Instructions) of the exercise. And Challenge Variations are just that, variations that increase the challenge of the Baseline Variation.

The order of the variations does not, necessarily, indicate increasing levels of difficulty; in many instances the variations are simply different, each designed to address a different need of the student. So Challenge Variation 4 may, or may not, be more challenging for you/your student than Challenge Variation 3. Note carefully the purpose noted for the variations. Just as not every exercise is suitable for every person, neither is every variation. As your/your student's mat routine continues to evolve over the months and years, continually evaluate what the body needs and choose thoughtfully the appropriate variation (Building, Baseline, or Challenge) of each exercise.

2. ABOUT THIS STUDY GUIDE

KATHI SUGGESTED at a workshop in 2016 that the way to get a glimpse into how she thinks of the Pilates repertoire was to go through her Mat book one exercise per week, in their *Add Next* order. That seemed like a great idea for a Facebook forum, which I started (the KRN Red Thread Reader's Group, if you're not a member yet please come join us - search Facebook for "KRN Red Thread Reader's Group" or go directly to the group at https://www.facebook.com/groups/KRNRedThreadReaders/).

Using the format of the Facebook forum as my guide I created this Study Guide to facilitate exploring Kathi's book at your own pace.

Here's the premise: Take one week to study one exercise. Do the variations in order - the Building Variations first, then the Baseline Variation (the Goal Instructions), then Challenge Variations, taking notice of the differences in each variation and why you would choose a particular variation over another for yourself, or for a student.

You have all week to explore these variations so take your time. Be mindful of any injuries or limitations. Respect where you are in your Pilates practice. Use your common sense and refer to the Injuries and Issues charts in the back on Kathi's book for Omit/Adjust recommendations for any issue(s) you/your student may have.

Teachers, treat yourself as your most valued client, there's no prize for doing any variation that you aren't ready for, or which isn't right for your body. Not being able to do every variation of an exercise? It's where most of us are and I call that practicing Pilates. On the other hand, it's good to have goals. So, if a variation is out of reach today make a plan using the *threads* to chart a logical course towards it.

As you get familiar with the variations and start to teach them to students, strive to choose the appropriate variation for that body. Identify what they need to build or challenge in that exercise and find the variation, or perhaps an exercise elsewhere in the studio, to facilitate that change.

When you're introducing exercises in one order but performing them in another, it can get confusing trying to see how all those pieces fit together. And the concept of a Performance Order may be new for some teachers. In the Classical Pilates world the mat repertoire is always done in the same order. Not every exercise is done, but the exercise that *are* done are done in the same order each time. The Mat repertoire is not a random list of exercises. And just as each exercise has a sequence to its individual movements, the Mat workout as a whole has a particular order. Complete lists of the full Foundational, Core and Advanced level mat exercise sequences, "The Order of Things", are on page 322 of *The Red Thread*©. As you build your/your student's mat routine one exercise at a time, it will fall in a particular place in the overall sequence. For each exercise I have noted the new Performance Order showing all the exercises up to that point with the new exercise in **BOLD.** Since many students will have a slightly different path to building their mat work, use the noted Performance Order as a guideline. If the Performance Order chart contains an exercise that you've not yet added to your/your student's mat routine simply leave it out, but do not change the sequence of the exercises that remain.

The tendency for many of us is to rush through. But give yourself that full week, or more, to feel the different variations, to start seeing that one exercise echo elsewhere in the Method. It's human nature to lose your momentum and we're talking about maybe a year long, or more, process to work through this book. So, have a plan. If you're teaching in a studio with other teachers, set aside a weekly meeting to explore the different variations and the hands on teaching suggestions; discuss what you would see in that exercise, or another exercise in the studio, that would lead you to choose a particular variation. If you have a break between clients, go back and forth between that that week's Mat exercise and the exercises listed in the "Connections to the Reformer" section (thank you Sunni Almond for that suggestion). Keep the book handy during your Mat workouts and take an extra few minutes to delve deeper in the exercise-of-the-week. In the back of this Study Guide you'll find a Progression Checklist listing all the variations. Use it to track your journey as you explore your way through the book. And we all get off track sometimes or need time for new information to soak in. If you need to take a break don't despair, just jump back in where you left off.

Most of all have fun. Because, as Kathi says, "Pilates should be fun – otherwise why bother doing it?"

3. INDEXES AND TABLES

THE FOLLOWING PAGES are indexes and tables I've built for myself. I hope you find them useful.

First is an alphabetical index for *The Red Thread*© so you can quickly find a specific exercise. Next is the list of exercises in their Add Next order. As Kathi stresses, these are just guidelines, but it's a handy reference table even so. Finally are tables for each individual *thread*. Note, the page numbers on all of these tables are not for this Study Guide, but are for *The Red Thread*© (RT).

The Red Thread of Pilates: The Mat©
Index by Exercise Name

EXERCISE NAME	RT PAGE #
Assisted Teaser 1	201
Assisted Teaser 2	205
Assisted Teaser 3	207
Assisted Teaser 4	211
Boomerang	265
Can Can	227
Control Balance	279
Corkscrew Flat	97
Corkscrew Full	103
Corkscrew Tail Off	101
Corkscrew Twist	105
Crab	275
Criss Cross	77
Double Leg Kick Back	125
Double Leg Pull Bent	63
Double Leg Straight	73
High Bicycle	143
High Bridge	291
High Scissors	141
Hip Circles	229
Hundred	29
Introduction to Neck Pull	133
Introduction to Open Leg Rocker	89
Introduction to Push Up	283
Jackknife	155
Kneeling Side Kicks - Bicycle	249
Kneeling Side Kicks - Circles	247
Kneeling Side Kicks - Front & Back	241
Kneeling Side Kicks - Up & Down	245
Leg Pull Back	239
Leg Pull Front	237
Mermaid	253
Neck Pull	135
Neck Roll	113
Open Leg Rocker	91
Pilates Push Up	285
Rocking	277
Roll Like a Ball	55
Roll Over	41
Roll Up	35
Saw	109
Seal With Beats	273

The Red Thread of Pilates: The Mat©
Index by Exercise Name

Exercises by Order of Introduction ("Add Next")

ADD NEXT	NAME	THREADS	RT PAGE
1	Hundred	S1	29
2	Roll Up	A1	35
3	Single Leg Circle	S2	45
4	Roll Like a Ball	R1	55
5	Single Leg Pull Bent	S3	59
6	Double Leg Pull Bent	S4	63
7	Spine Stretch Forward	A2	83
8	Seal Without Beats	R2	271
9	Single Leg Pull Straight	S5	69
10	Assisted Teaser 1	A3	201
11	Assisted Teaser 2	A4	205
12	Assisted Teaser 3	A5	207
13	Assisted Teaser 4	A6	211
14	Single Leg Kick Back	S6, E1	121
15	Saw	T1	109
16	Introduction to Push Up	S7, [A6+]	283
17	Introduction to Open Leg Rocker	S8	89
18	Open Leg Rocker	R3	91
19	Introduction to Neck Pull	A7	133
PRE 20	Side Kicks – Set Up & Focus	[S]	159
20	Side Kicks - Up & Down	S9, SB1	167
21	Side Kicks - Front & Back	S10, E2	163
22	Side Kicks - Small Circles	S11, SB2, E3	169
23	Single Leg Tick Tock	T2	51
24	Double Leg Straight	S12	73
25	Criss Cross	T3	77
26	Corkscrew Flat	T4	97
27	Neck Roll	T5, E4	113
28	Teaser 1	A8	215
29	Double Leg Kick Back	S13, E5	125
30	Single Leg Circle Full	T6	53
31	Neck Pull	A9	135
32	Corkscrew Tail Off	T7	101
33	Side Kicks - Bicycle	S14, E6	189
34	Seal With Beats	R4	273
35	Can Can	T8	227
36	Pilates Push Up	S15, [A9+]	285
37	Side Kick - Medium Circles	S16, SB3, E7	171
38	Swan Preparation	S17, E8	115
39	Mermaid	SB4	253
40	Spine Twist	T9	151
41	Teaser 2	S18	219
42	Side Kicks - Inner Thigh Lifts	S19	175

Exercises by Order of Introduction ("Add Next")

ADD NEXT	NAME	THREADS	RT PAGE
43	Side Kicks - Inner Thigh Circle	S20	177
44	Side Kicks - Side Bicycle	S21, SB5	179
45	Side Kicks - Double Leg Lifts	S22, SB6	183
46	Side Kicks - Beats	S23, SB7	185
47	Side Kicks - Crosses	S24, SB8	187
48	Side Kicks - Large Circles	S25, SB9, E9	173
49	Corkscrew Full	T10	103
50	Swimming	S26, E10	233
51	Kneeling Side Kicks - Up & Down	S27, SB10	245
52	Kneeling Side Kicks - Front & Back	S28, E11	241
53	Side Kicks - Grand Circles	S29, E12, SB11	193
54	Roll Over	A10	41
55	Teaser 3	A11	221
56	Hip Circles	T11	229
57	Leg Pull Front	S30, E13	237
58	Leg Pull Back	S31, E14	239
59	Thigh Stretch	S32	129
60	Side Bend	SB12	261
61	Snake & Twist	SB13, E15, T12, A12	257
62	Jackknife	A13	155
63	Corkscrew Twist	T13	105
64	Tick Tock	T14	107
65	Kneeling Side Kicks - Circles	S33, E16, SB14	247
66	Kneeling Side Kicks - Bicycle	S34, E17	249
67	Rocking	S35, E18, R5	277
68	Swan Dive	S36, E19, R6	119
69	Control Balance	S37	279
70	Shoulder Bridge	S38, E20	147
71	Side Kicks - Hot Potato	S39, SB15	197
72	Side Kicks - Big Scissors	S40, E21	199
73	Boomerang	R7	265
74	High Scissors	S41, E22	141
75	High Bicycle	S42, E23	143
76	Crab	R8	275
77	High Bridge	S43, E24	291

[mine, not KRN]

Stability Thread

ADD NEXT	NAME	THREAD #	RT PAGE
1	Hundred	S1	29
3	Single Leg Circle	S2	45
5	Single Leg Pull Bent	S3	59
6	Double Leg Pull Bent	S4	63
9	Single Leg Pull Straight	S5	69
14	Single Leg Kick Back	S6	121
16	Introduction to Push Up	S7	283
17	Introduction to Open Leg Rocker	S8	89
PRE 20	Side Kicks – Set Up & Focus	[S9 prep]	159
20	Side Kicks - Up & Down	S9	167
21	Side Kicks - Front & Back	S10	163
22	Side Kicks - Small Circles	S11	169
24	Double Leg Straight	S12	73
29	Double Leg Kick Back	S13	125
33	Side Kicks - Bicycle	S14	189
36	Pilates Push Up	S15	285
37	Side Kicks - Medium Circles	S16	171
38	Swan Preparation	S17	115
41	Teaser 2	S18	219
42	Side Kicks - Inner Thigh Lifts	S19	175
43	Side Kicks - Inner Thigh Circle	S20	177
44	Side Kicks - Side Bicycle	S21	179
45	Side Kicks - Double Leg Lifts	S22	183
46	Side Kicks - Beats	S23	185
47	Side Kicks - Crosses	S24	187
48	Side Kicks - Large Circles	S25	173
50	Swimming	S26	233
51	Kneeling Side Kicks - Up & Down	S27	245
52	Kneeling Side Kicks - Front & Back	S28	241
53	Side Kicks - Grand Circles	S29	193
57	Leg Pull Front	S30	237
58	Leg Pull Back	S31	239
59	Thigh Stretch	S32	129
66	Kneeling Side Kicks - Bicycle	S34	249
67	Rocking	S35	277
68	Swan Dive	S36	119
69	Control Balance	S37	279
70	Shoulder Bridge	S38	147
71	Side Kicks - Hot Potato	S39	197
72	Side Kicks - Big Scissors	S40	199
74	High Scissors	S41	141
75	High Bicycle	S42	143
77	High Bridge	S43	291

Articulation Thread

ADD NEXT	NAME	THREAD #	RT PAGE
2	Roll Up	A1	35
7	Spine Stretch Forward	A2	83
10	Assisted Teaser 1	A3	201
11	Assisted Teaser 2	A4	205
12	Assisted Teaser 3	A5	207
13	Assisted Teaser 4	A6	211
*16	Introduction to the Push Up	A6+	283
19	Introduction to Neck Pull	A7	133
28	Teaser 1	A8	215
31	Neck Pull	A9	135
*36	Pilates Push Up	A9+	285
54	Roll Over	A10	41
55	Teaser 3	A11	221
61	Snake & Twist	A12	257
62	Jackknife	A13	155

* Mine, not KRN

Rolling Thread

ADD NEXT	NAME	THREAD #	RT PAGE
4	Roll Like a Ball	RF1	55
8	Seal Without Beats	RF2	271
18	Open Leg Rocker	RF3	91
34	Seal With Beats	RF4	273
67	Rocking	RE5	277
68	Swan Dive	RE6	119
73	Boomerang	RF7	265
76	Crab	RF8	275

Extension Thread

ADD NEXT	NAME	THREAD #	RT PAGE
14	Single Leg Kick Back	E1	121
21	Side Kicks - Front & Back	E2	163
22	Side Kicks - Small Circles	E3	169
27	Neck Roll	E4	113
29	Double Leg Kick Back	E5	125
33	Side Kicks - Bicycle	E6	189
37	Side Kicks - Medium Circles	E7	171
38	Swan Preparation	E8	115
48	Side Kicks - Large Circles	E9	173
50	Swimming	E10	233
52	Kneeling Side Kicks - Front & Back	E11	241
53	Side Kicks - Grand Circles	E12	193
57	Leg Pull Front	E13	237
58	Leg Pull Back	E14	239
61	Snake & Twist	E15	257
65	Kneeling Side Kicks - Circles	E16	247
66	Kneeling Side Kicks - Bicycle	E17	249
67	Rocking	E18	277
68	Swan Dive	E19	119
70	Shoulder Bridge	E20	147
72	Side Kicks - Big Scissors	E21	199
74	High Scissors	E22	141
75	High Bicycle	E23	143
77	High Bridge	E24	291

Twisting Thread

ADD NEXT	NAME	THREAD #	RT PAGE
15	Saw	T1	109
23	Single Leg Tick Tock	T2	51
25	Criss Cross	T3	77
26	Corkscrew Flat	T4	97
27	Neck Roll	T5	113
30	Single Leg Circle Full	T6	53
32	Corkscrew Tail Off	T7	101
35	Can Can	T8	227
40	Spine Twist	T9	151
49	Corkscrew Full	T10	103
56	Hip Circles	T11	229
61	Snake & Twist	T12	257
63	Corkscrew Twist	T13	105
64	Tick Tock	T14	107

Side Bending Thread

ADD NEXT	NAME	THREAD #	RT PAGE
20	Side Kicks - Up & Down	SB1	167
22	Side Kicks - Small Circles	SB2	169
37	Side Kicks - Medium Circles	SB3	171
39	Mermaid	SB4	253
44	Side Kicks - Side Bicycle	SB5	179
45	Side Kicks - Double Leg Lifts	SB6	183
46	Side Kicks - Beats	SB7	185
47	Side Kicks - Crosses	SB8	187
48	Side Kicks - Large Circles	SB9	173
51	Kneeling Side Kicks - Up & Down	SB10	245
53	Side Kicks - Grand Circles	SB11	193
60	Side Bend	SB12	261
61	Snake & Twist	SB13	257
65	Kneeling Side Kicks - Circles	SB14	247
71	Side Kicks - Hot Potato	SB15	197

4. THE EXERCISES

THE FOLLOWING PAGES are worksheets for each exercise, in their *Add Next* order.

If Kathi has noted a particular purpose for a variation it will be noted below the Variation in *italics*. These are often annotated. Please always refer to *The Red Thread©* for complete descriptions.

The Performance Order noted after each exercise assumes the mat workout is being constructed in the *Add Next* order. However, since the Add Next order is simply a guideline, it is likely that the Performance Order for any individual will be slightly different because some exercises have not yet been added to their mat workout. If the Performance Order includes an exercise that has not been added to someone's mat routine, simply leave it out, but do not change the sequence of the other exercises.

The Red Thread® is all about connections, how the Pilates repertoire is threaded together, using one exercise to prepare the body for another, perhaps on another apparatus. For each exercise, Kathi details the connections of that exercise to the prior exercise of the thread, and to the prior exercise in the Performance Order, and lists the related exercises on the Reformer and the Mat. But connections are also woven through the variations. Some variations are essentially Building Variations for a completely different exercise so pay particular attention to those purposes that refer to another exercise. Also be on the lookout for recommendations of exercises on other apparatus and hands on spotting options in the Teaching notes for each exercises. Don't get so dazzled by all the variations that you miss the intricate web of how they are all connected to the rest of the repertoire – that, for me, is where the magic lies.

Enough talk. Ready to move?

The Hundred

Add Next	1
Pages	29-34
Thread(s)	Stability 1

Foundational:

- Building Variation 1: Legs Flat on The Mat, Feet Under Strap
  To introduce Hundred.
- Building Variation 2: Barrel
  To support upper back if needed to find correct upper back position.

Core:

- Building Variation 3: Single Leg Lift & Lower
  To build Powerhouse to hold weight of legs.
- Building Variation 4: Single Leg Lower & Lift
  To build Powerhouse to hold weight of legs and increase lower stomach strength.
- Building Variation 5: Double Leg Lower & Lift
  To build Powerhouse to hold weight of legs and pelvic stability. Enables you to find range of motion.
- Building Variation 6: Parallel Lines
  To connect the upper and lower body. Helps to build complete abdominal strength and connects arms to back.
- Baseline Version: Goal Instructions

Advanced:

- Challenge Variation 7: Heel Beats
  To challenge pelvic stability and tone inner thighs.
- Challenge Variation 8: Walking
  To challenge Powerhouse, work back of legs and develop pelvic stability.
- Challenge Variation 9: Weighted Bar
  To challenge upper stomach and deepen connection to Powerhouse. Helps to open chest and lower back.

**The Order of Things
after The Hundred**

PERFORMANCE ORDER	EXERCISE	ADD NEXT #
1	**HUNDRED**	1

The Roll Up

Add Next	2
Pages	35-40
Thread(s)	Articulation 1

Foundational:
- Building Variation 1: Roll Up - Hand Slide
  To build and isolate upper stomach strength.
- Building Variation 2: Roll Back
  To build lower stomach strength.
- Building Variation 3: Roll Down
  Use to increase spinal opening after the Roll Back Variation is mastered.
- Building Variation 4: Speed Bump
  To prevent the upper back from touching the Mat before the lower back. Note: this can be used with any variation.
- Building Variation 5: Teacher Holds Bar
  To help connect to Powerhouse and open lower back.

Core:
- Building Variation 6: Hook the Foot
  To open lower back and for student who stretches too far forward.
- Building Variation 7: Hand Slide on Full Roll Up
  Use for student who rounds upper back or for student who "dolphins" over and has "C-Curve" in upper back and not lower back.
- Baseline Version: Goal Instructions

Advanced:
- Challenge Variation 8: Roll Up with Pointed Feet
  For the strong student who grips with their legs.
- Challenge Variation 9: Pause
  To strengthen and clarify weaker point.
- Challenge Variation 10: Up Two – Down One
  To challenge strength and articulation
- Challenge Variation 11: Wide Grip
  To challenge articulation.

The Order of Things
after The Roll Up

PERFORMANCE ORDER	EXERCISE	ADD NEXT #
1	Hundred	1
2	**ROLL UP**	**2**

Single Leg Circle

Add Next	3
Pages	45-49
Thread(s)	Stability 2

Foundational:

- Building Variation 1: Bent Knee – Sign of The Cross
  To build knowledge of center and where to move the leg.
- Building Variation 2: Bent Knee – Small Circles
  Helps with pelvic stability; use for sway backs, and larger bottoms.
- Building Variation 3: Small Circles with Bent Base Knee
  Helps with pelvic stability; use for sway backs, and larger bottoms; to stretch back of leg.
- Building Variation 4: Small Circles with Wide Base
  Use for a pelvis that wobbles.
- Baseline Variation: Goal Instructions through step 10

Core:

- Add Single Leg Tick Tock (*Add Next #23*) for last 2-3 circles on each side (Goal Instructions through step 11)

Advanced:

- Replace Single Leg Tick Tock with Single Leg Circle Full (*Add Next #30*) for the last two circles on each side (Goal Instructions through step 12)

Super Advanced:

- Challenge Variation 5: Arm Overhead with Weights
  To challenge torso stability.
- Challenge Variation 6: Lifted Bottom Leg
  To challenge Powerhouse and control.

The Order of Things
after Single Leg Circle

PERFORMANCE ORDER	EXERCISE	ADD NEXT #
1	Hundred	1
2	Roll Up	2
3	**SINGLE LEG CIRCLE**	3

Roll Like a Ball

Add Next	4
Pages	55-58
Thread(s)	Rolling (Forward) 1

Foundational:
- Building Variation 1: Roll Back
  Use this variation if Student is unable to Roll (Building Variation 2 of The Roll Up).
- Baseline Variation: Goal Instructions

Core:
- Challenge Variation 2: Full Roll to Shoulders
  Increases spinal massage throughout entire spine.
- Challenge Variation 3: Accent
  Works breath and stomach. This variation introduces dynamic action.

Advanced:
- Challenge Variation 4: Advanced Hand Position
  Increases abdominal work and decreases movement available to cheat.
- Challenge Variation 5: Hold and Balance
  To increase balance; teach in preparation for Open Leg Rocker.
- Challenge Variation 6: Shoulder Stand into Roll
  To increases control and balance; teach in preparation for Control Balance and Boomerang.
- Challenge Variation 7: Teaser into Roll
  To increase control and abdominal work; teach in preparation for Boomerang.
- Challenge Variation 8: Teaser Shoulder Stand Combo
  To increase control, balance and abdominal work. Increases dynamic movement.
- Challenge Variation 9: Roll to Stand
  To add dynamic movement and connection to propulsion. This is a great preparation before introducing the Russian on the Reformer.
- Challenge Variation 10: Roll to Jump
  To add dynamic movement and connects to propulsion. This is a great preparation before introducing the Russian on the Reformer.
- Challenge Variation 11: Stand with Single Leg Front
  To challenge balance and strengthen legs. Preps for Russian on the Reformer.

- Challenge Variation 12: Stand with Single Leg Front into Kneeling Knee Scale on Foot into Backbend
  Requires more balance and opens hips. Teach in preparation for Russian One Leg Squats on Reformer.
- Challenge Variation 13: Single Leg Russian Roll
  To add dynamic movement and connect it to propulsion. A great preparation before introducing the Russian on the Reformer.
- Challenge Variation 14: Elbows to Knees
  Use for the strong student who muscles with arm and upper body.

The Order of Things
after Roll Like a Ball

PERFORMANCE ORDER	EXERCISE	ADD NEXT #
1	Hundred	1
2	Roll Up	2
3	Single Leg Circle	3
4	**ROLL LIKE A BALL**	**4**

Single Leg Pull Bent

Add Next	5
Pages	59-62
Thread(s)	Stability 3

Foundational:
- Building Variation 1: Change with Two Legs into Chest
  Use as an introduction to focus on pelvic stability.
- Building Variation 2: Fluid Change
  To hone the coordination of moving two sides in opposition with a stable Box.
- Baseline Variation: Goal Instructions

Core:
- Challenge Variation 3: Teaser Change
  Introduces the Teaser.

Advanced:
- Increase reps to 10 (5 each leg)
- Challenge Variation 4: Extended Leg Pause
  Teach prior to introducing Teaser 1
- Challenge Variation 5: Slice off Bottom (Bicycle)
  To trim the bottom and challenge the stability of the pelvis. Introduce this variation prior to learning Bicycle in the Side Kicks.
- Challenge Variation 6: No Hands
  For carpal tunnel, hand, elbow, wrist and shoulder issues. Also can be used to challenge the Powerhouse.

Super Advanced:
- Challenge Variation 7: Rolling Up into Teaser
  To develop the musculature needed for smooth transitions on the Reformer.

The Order of Things
after Single Leg Pull Bent

PERFORMANCE ORDER	EXERCISE	ADD NEXT #
1	Hundred	1
2	Roll Up	2
3	Single Leg Circle	3
4	Roll Like a Ball	4
5	**SINGLE LEG PULL BENT**	**5**

Double Leg Pull Bent

Foundational:

- Building Variation 1: Arms by Sides
  Use as an introduction. Also helps keep the Box square for students who like to shorten one side.
- Building Variation 2: Hand Slide on Legs
  For the student who drops their feet while the knees return to the chest.

Core:

- Building Variation 3: Arms Straight Back & In
  To increase the coordination challenge and increase depth of the inhale and exhale.
- Building Variation 4: No Hands
  For carpal tunnel, hand, elbow, wrist and shoulder issues. Hands may be placed by side on Mat if support is needed.
  Note: this appears to be the same as Building Variation 1.
- Baseline Variation: Goal Instructions

Advanced:

- Challenge Variation 5: Back Stroke
  To build abdominal strength and coordination.
- Challenge Variation 6: Count Hold Arm Circles
  To increase coordination, control and an understanding of how rhythm affects movement.
- Challenge Variation 7: Fully Open
  Use in preparation for the introduction of Teaser 3.
- Challenge Variation 8: Backstroke Swimming
- Challenge Variation 9: Around the Clock
  To build the coordination needed for transitions on the Reformer.

**The Order of Things
after Double Leg Pull Bent**

PERFORMANCE ORDER	EXERCISE	ADD NEXT #
1	Hundred	1
2	Roll Up	2
3	Single Leg Circle	3
4	Roll Like a Ball	4
5	Single Leg Pull Bent	5
6	**DOUBLE LEG PULL BENT**	**6**

Spine Stretch Forward

Add Next	7
Pages	83-87
Thread(s)	Articulation 2

Foundational:

- Building Variation 1: Walk Hands
  Use to introduce the Spine Stretch Forward. Helps to prevent overstretching and maintains the focus on opening the lower back.
- Building Variation 2: Slide Hands Along Legs
  To open the lower back and prevent student from stretching too far forward.
- Building Variation 3: Grab and Pull
  Do this variation before introducing Introduction to Open Leg Rocker.
- Building Variation 4: Alternating Bend of Knee
  To increase the stretch in the back of the leg.
- Building Variation 5: Bend Both Knees
  To increase the stretch in the back of the leg.
- Baseline Variation: Goal Instructions

Core:

- Challenge Variation 7: Arm Circles
  Use to add a chest opening.
- Challenge Variation 8: Rowing Arms
  To open the chest and shoulders.

Advanced:

- Challenge Variation 9: Pulses
  To deepen the stretch throughout the body.
- Challenge Variation 10: Diagonal – Flat Back
  For the student who likes to round forward or sit back.

The Order of Things
after Spine Stretch Forward

PERFORMANCE ORDER	EXERCISE	ADD NEXT #
1	Hundred	1
2	Roll Up	2
3	Single Leg Circle	3
4	Roll Like a Ball	4
5	Single Leg Pull Bent	5
6	Double Leg Pull Bent	6
7	**SPINE STRETCH FORWARD**	**7**

Seal Without Beats

Add Next	8
Pages	271-272
Thread(s)	Rolling (Forward) 2

No Variations

Foundational:

- Baseline Variation: Goal Instructions

Core Level +: Replace with Seal With Beats (Add Next #34)

**The Order of Things
after Seal Without Beats**

PERFORMANCE ORDER	EXERCISE	ADD NEXT #
1	Hundred	1
2	Roll Up	2
3	Single Leg Circle	3
4	Roll Like a Ball	4
5	Single Leg Pull Bent	5
6	Double Leg Pull Bent	6
7	Spine Stretch Forward	7
8	**SEAL WITHOUT BEATS**	**8**

Single Leg Pull Straight

Add Next	9
Pages	69-71
Thread(s)	Stability 5

Foundational:
- Building Variation 1: Change with Legs Up
  Use as an introduction to focus on pelvic stability.
- Building Variation 2: Fluid Switch
  To hone the coordination of moving two sides in opposition with a stable box. Great to build stability needed for Side Kick Series.
- Baseline Variation: Goal Instructions

Core:
- Challenge Variation 4: Hands by Side
  Great variation for carpal tunnel, hand, elbow, wrist and shoulder issues. Also can be used to challenge the Powerhouse.

Advanced:
- Increase repetitions to 10 (5 each leg)
- Challenge Variation 5: Upper Body Lifted
  Great variation for hypermobile people and for people who don't use their entire stomach to support the Powerhouse.
- Challenge Variation 6: Roll Up
  To develop the musculature needed for smooth transitions on the Reformer.

Note: This is the first instance of the Performance Order (the sequence in which the exercises are performed) and the Add Next Number (the sequence in which the exercises are added to the workout) being different. Single Leg Pull Straight is the 9th exercise taught to the client (Add Next #9) but it's inserted into the Performance Order after the Double Leg Pull Bent and before Spine Stretch Forward. This will be the usual case from here on out, that the next exercise to be added to the mat workout gets inserted within the Performance Order. The newly added exercise will always be **bolded** in the Performance Order chart.

The Order of Things
after Single Leg Pull Straight

PERFORMANCE ORDER	EXERCISE	ADD NEXT #
1	Hundred	1
2	Roll Up	2
3	Single Leg Circle	3
4	Roll Like a Ball	4
5	Single Leg Pull Bent	5
6	Double Leg Pull Bent	6
7	**SINGLE LEG PULL STRAIGHT**	**9**
8	Spine Stretch Forward	7
9	Seal Without Beats	8

Assisted Teaser 1
Half Way Up

Add Next	10
Pages	201-203
Thread(s)	Articulation 3

Foundational 2:
- Baseline Variation: Goal Instructions
    - Spotting Variation 1: Hold Hands
    To create resistance for student to scoop against as they roll down, until the understanding of self-resistance or Two Way Stretch is learned.
    - Spotting Variation 2: Hold Ankles
    To aid in resistance and prevent the feet from moving.
    - Spotting Variation 3: Reach for Shoulders
- Challenge Variation 1: Arms by Ears
- Challenge Variation 2: Half Way Down

Core Level +: Replace with Teaser 1

The Order of Things
after Assisted Teaser 1

PERFORMANCE ORDER	EXERCISE	ADD NEXT #
1	Hundred	1
2	Roll Up	2
3	Single Leg Circle	3
4	Roll Like a Ball	4
5	Single Leg Pull Bent	5
6	Double Leg Pull Bent	6
7	Single Leg Pull Straight	9
8	Spine Stretch Forward	7
9	**ASSISTED TEASER 1**	**10**
10	Seal Without Beats	8

Assisted Teaser 2
One Leg Up

Add Next	11
Pages	205-206
Thread(s)	Articulation 4

Foundational 2:
- Baseline Variation: Goal Instructions
  - Spotting Variation 1: Hold Hands
    To aid and create resistance.
  - Spotting Variation 2: Hold Leg
    To aid in resistance and prevent the foot from moving.
  - Spotting Variation 3: Reach for Shoulders
- Challenge Variation 1: Single Leg Twist

Core Level +: Replace with Teaser 1

The Order of Things
after Assisted Teaser 2

PERFORMANCE ORDER	EXERCISE	ADD NEXT #
1	Hundred	1
2	Roll Up	2
3	Single Leg Circle	3
4	Roll Like a Ball	4
5	Single Leg Pull Bent	5
6	Double Leg Pull Bent	6
7	Single Leg Pull Straight	9
8	Spine Stretch Forward	7
9	Assisted Teaser 1	10
10	**ASSISTED TEASER 2**	**11**
11	Seal Without Beats	8

Assisted Teaser 3
Hold Wrist

Add Next	12
Pages	207-209
Thread(s)	Articulation 5

Foundational 2:

- Building Variation 1: Half Way Down
- Baseline Variation: Goal Instructions
- Challenge Variation 3: Single Leg Fully Up
  This variation is Assisted Teaser 2 (One Leg Up) plus the full Roll Up of
  Assisted Teaser 3. No spotter is required. *Use to challenge stability.*
- Challenge Variation 4: Legs Up Twist
  Use to increase stability when twisting.

Core Level +: Replace with Teaser 1

This exercise requires a spotter. Omit if practicing without a teacher.

The Order of Things
after Assisted Teaser 3

PERFORMANCE ORDER	EXERCISE	ADD NEXT #
1	Hundred	1
2	Roll Up	2
3	Single Leg Circle	3
4	Roll Like a Ball	4
5	Single Leg Pull Bent	5
6	Double Leg Pull Bent	6
7	Single Leg Pull Straight	9
8	Spine Stretch Forward	7
9	Assisted Teaser 1	10
10	Assisted Teaser 2	11
11	**ASSISTED TEASER 3***	**12**
12	Seal Without Beats	8

*requires a spotter; omit if none

Assisted Teaser 4
Hold Toes

Add Next	13
Pages	211-213
Thread(s)	Articulation 6

Foundational 2:

- Building Variation 1: Half Way Down
- Building Variation 2: Feet on Thighs – Down to Full Up
  Use to build to the full Teaser 1
- Baseline Variation: Goal Instructions
- Challenge Variation 3: Arms by Ears
- Challenge Variation 4: Twist

Core Level +: Replace with Teaser 1

This exercises requires a spotter. Omit if practicing without a teacher.

The Order of Things
after Assisted Teaser 4

PERFORMANCE ORDER	EXERCISE	ADD NEXT #
1	Hundred	1
2	Roll Up	2
3	Single Leg Circle	3
4	Roll Like a Ball	4
5	Single Leg Pull Bent	5
6	Double Leg Pull Bent	6
7	Single Leg Pull Straight	9
8	Spine Stretch Forward	7
9	Assisted Teaser 1	10
10	Assisted Teaser 2	11
11	Assisted Teaser 3*	12
12	**ASSISTED TEASER 4***	**13**
13	Seal Without Beats	8

*requires a spotter; omit if none

Single Leg Kick Back

Add Next	14
Pages	121-124
Thread(s)	Stability 6
	Extension 1

Foundational:

- Building Variation 1: Diaper
Preparation for all work on the stomach.
- Baseline Variation: Goal Instructions

Core:

- Challenge Variation 2: Single Leg Thighs Off Mat
To work the bottom and increase the two way stretch.
- Challenge Variation 3: Flex and Point
To improve coordination and stretch the calf.

Advanced:

- Challenge Variation 4: Both Thighs Off
To work the bottom.

The Order of Things
after Single Leg Kick Back

PERFORMANCE ORDER	EXERCISE	ADD NEXT #
1	Hundred	1
2	Roll Up	2
3	Single Leg Circle	3
4	Roll Like a Ball	4
5	Single Leg Pull Bent	5
6	Double Leg Pull Bent	6
7	Single Leg Pull Straight	9
8	Spine Stretch Forward	7
9	**SINGLE LEG KICK BACK**	**14**
10	Assisted Teaser 1	10
11	Assisted Teaser 2	11
12	Assisted Teaser 3*	12
13	Assisted Teaser 4*	13
14	Seal Without Beats	8

*requires a spotter; omit if none

The Saw

Add Next	15
Pages	109-112
Thread(s)	Twisting 1

Foundational 2:

- Building Variation 1: Side Bend with Bent Arms
  To introduce Saw and for the student who lifts the opposite hip.
- Building Variation 2: Side Bend into Twist
  To introduce the Twist and for the student who likes to shorten one side while twisting.
- Baseline Variation: Goal Instructions

Core:

- Move fluidly through each position

Advanced:

- Challenge Variation 3: Full Twist
  To add full rotation through the upper body. Teach this when you add one-legged Elephant with a Twist on the Reformer, and before Snake and Twist.
- Challenge Variation 4: Open Chest
  For the student who collapses the chest during the Twist or needs more chest opening.

The Order of Things
after The Saw

PERFORMANCE ORDER	EXERCISE	ADD NEXT #
1	Hundred	1
2	Roll Up	2
3	Single Leg Circle	3
4	Roll Like a Ball	4
5	Single Leg Pull Bent	5
6	Double Leg Pull Bent	6
7	Single Leg Pull Straight	9
8	Spine Stretch Forward	7
9	**SAW**	**15**
10	Single Leg Kick Back	14
11	Assisted Teaser 1	10
12	Assisted Teaser 2	11
13	Assisted Teaser 3*	12
14	Assisted Teaser 4*	13
15	Seal Without Beats	8

*requires a spotter; omit if none

Introduction to The Push Up

Add Next	16
Pages	283-284
Thread(s)	Stability 7 [Articulation]

No variations

Foundational 2:

* Baseline Variation: Goal Instructions
  Teaching note: Teach this before the Long Stretch Series on the Reformer.

Core Level +: Replace with The Push Up (Add Next #36)

Kathi does not include this as part of the Articulation Thread, but it belongs there, in my opinion. The spine articulates to get into the plank position and Kathi uses the "a- word" in Instruction 2: "Articulate the spine down, as if you are doing a standing Roll Up".

The Order of Things
after Introduction to the Push Up

PERFORMANCE ORDER	EXERCISE	ADD NEXT #
1	Hundred	1
2	Roll Up	2
3	Single Leg Circle	3
4	Roll Like a Ball	4
5	Single Leg Pull Bent	5
6	Double Leg Pull Bent	6
7	Single Leg Pull Straight	9
8	Spine Stretch Forward	7
9	Saw	15
10	Single Leg Kick Back	14
11	Assisted Teaser 1	10
12	Assisted Teaser 2	11
13	Assisted Teaser 3*	12
14	Assisted Teaser 4*	13
15	Seal Without Beats	8
16	**INTRODUCTION TO THE PUSH UP**	**16**

*requires a spotter; omit if none

Introduction to Open Leg Rocker

Add Next	17
Pages	89-90
Thread(s)	Stability 8

Foundational 2:

- Building Variation 1: Double Leg Extension
  Use this variation to introduce the Open Leg Rocker and to build balance.
- Building Variation 2: Open & Close
  To challenge balance.
- Baseline Variation: Goal Instructions

Core Level +: Replace with Open Leg Rocker (Add Next #18)

The Order of Things
after Introduction to Open Leg Rocker

PERFORMANCE ORDER	EXERCISE	ADD NEXT #
1	Hundred	1
2	Roll Up	2
3	Single Leg Circle	3
4	Roll Like a Ball	4
5	Single Leg Pull Bent	5
6	Double Leg Pull Bent	6
7	Single Leg Pull Straight	9
8	Spine Stretch Forward	7
9	**INTRODUCTION TO OPEN LEG ROCKER**	**17**
10	Saw	15
11	Single Leg Kick Back	14
12	Assisted Teaser 1	10
13	Assisted Teaser 2	11
14	Assisted Teaser 3*	12
15	Assisted Teaser 4*	13
16	Seal Without Beats	8
17	Introduction to the Push Up	16

*requires a spotter; omit if none

Open Leg Rocker

Add Next	18
Pages	91-95
Thread(s)	Rolling (Forward) 3

Foundational 2:
- Baseline Variation: Goal Instructions
- Challenge Variation 1: Toe Touch
  To increase spinal massage. Teach in preparation for rolling over to stand (Challenge Variation 9).

Advanced:
- Challenge Variation 2: Closed Leg Rocker – Big Toes
  To increase the stretch of the back of the leg and opening of the lower back. This is a great preparation for introducing the Teaser.
- Challenge Variation 3: Closed Leg Rocker – Little Toes
  To increase the stretch of the back of the leg and the opening of the lower back. Great for the student who likes to curl their little toes forward.
- Challenge Variation 4: Shave Stretch
  To add a deep stretch for the back of the legs and the spine. The student who needs the Tower stretch on the Cadillac can benefit from this stretch.
- Challenge Variation 5: Wide Leg Rocker
  To challenge the ability to roll as well as to stretch tight hips.
- Challenge Variation 6: Flat Hands – Legs Open
  Use for the student who likes to hang in or round their upper back when rolling.
- Challenge Variation 7: Flat Hands – Legs Closed
  Use for the student who likes to hang in or round their upper back when rolling.
- Challenge Variation 8: Open Leg Rocker Spine Stretch Combo
  Adds focus on controlling the legs as they lower. Great to teach in preparation for the Boomerang.
- Challenge Variation 9: Roll Back to Stand
  Teach after Roll Over has been taught. Note – usually placed after 3 Open Leg Rockers and 2 Closed Leg Rockers
- Challenge Variation 10: Roll Back to Stand with Backbend
  To utilize flexion and extension with control. Note – use as an ending to Open Leg Rocker.

- Challenge Variation 11: Open Leg Rocker/Spine Stretch to Stand Combo
To utilize full flexion and full extension with control. A combination of Spine Stretch Forward and Challenge Variation 1.

The Order of Things
after Open Leg Rocker

PERFORMANCE ORDER	EXERCISE	ADD NEXT #
1	Hundred	1
2	Roll Up	2
3	Single Leg Circle	3
4	Roll Like a Ball	4
5	Single Leg Pull Bent	5
6	Double Leg Pull Bent	6
7	Single Leg Pull Straight	9
8	Spine Stretch Forward	7
9	Introduction to Open Leg Rocker	17
10	**OPEN LEG ROCKER**	**18**
11	Saw	15
12	Single Leg Kick Back	14
13	Assisted Teaser 1	10
14	Assisted Teaser 2	11
15	Assisted Teaser 3*	12
16	Assisted Teaser 4*	13
17	Seal Without Beats	8
18	Introduction to the Push Up	16

*requires a spotter; omit if none

Introduction to The Neck Pull

Add Next	19
Pages	133-134
Thread(s)	Articulation 7

No official Variations but the Teaching tips contain these break downs:
- Draw elbows towards each other
  For students unable to roll up with elbows open.
- Hold back of legs at sticking point
  For students who get "stuck" rolling up or down.

Foundational 2:
- Baseline Variation: Goal Instructions

Core Level +: Replace with The Neck Pull (Add Next #31)

The Order of Things
after Introduction to Neck Pull

PERFORMANCE ORDER	EXERCISE	ADD NEXT #
1	Hundred	1
2	Roll Up	2
3	Single Leg Circle	3
4	Roll Like a Ball	4
5	Single Leg Pull Bent	5
6	Double Leg Pull Bent	6
7	Single Leg Pull Straight	9
8	Spine Stretch Forward	7
9	Introduction to Open Leg Rocker	17
10	Open Leg Rocker	18
11	Saw	15
12	Single Leg Kick Back	14
13	**INTRODUCTION TO NECK PULL**	**19**
14	Assisted Teaser 1	10
15	Assisted Teaser 2	11
16	Assisted Teaser 3*	12
17	Assisted Teaser 4*	13
18	Seal Without Beats	8
19	Introduction to the Push Up	16

*requires a spotter; omit if none

Side Kicks – Set Up & Focus

Add Next	Pre 20
Pages	159-162
Thread(s)	Stability

There is no Add Next number for this as it's not an exercise, per se, but it is clearly meant to be reviewed before you introduce the Side Kick series. Unless you're reading the book from cover to cover it's possible to miss these incredibly informative pages about teaching the Side Kick Series. Don't skip these pages, there's a lot of treasure to be found here!

Foundational:
- Building Variation 1: Arm Long & Head on Arm (with foot under strap)
  Introduce in this position.
- Baseline Variation 2: On Elbow
  To strengthen the side body and challenge balance.

Core:
- Challenge Variation 3: Remove Strap to Challenge Stability
  To bring awareness to the side against the Mat and increase understanding of the Two Way Stretch. Teach before introducing the Side Bend.
- Challenge Variation 4: Top Hand Behind Head
  To strengthen the side body and challenge balance. Teach before the Side Sit Up Series on the apparatus.

Advanced:
- Challenge Variation 5: Top Arm Along Side Body
  To challenge balance. Teach this before the Kneeling Side Kick Series.
- Challenge Variation 6: One Straight Line
  Teach this variation before teaching the Star on the Reformer.

Super Advanced:
- Challenge Variation 7: Add Light Ankle Weights
  To build the strength needed for the Star and Snake & Twist on the Reformer.
- Challenge Variation 8: Both Arms Reach Overhead
  Use as a preparation for the One Leg Side Sit Up Series on the apparatus.

Transition Options:

- Pre-transition option: See Challenge Variation 11 of Criss-Cross (*Add Next #25*) – Hip Lift/Bent Knee at 90-degrees or Straight Line
- Plain Transition
  To reset spinal alignment.
- Beat Transition
  To engage Trinity and reset spinal alignment.
- Split Change Transition

Side Kicks – Up & Down

Add Next	20
Pages	167-168
Thread(s)	Stability 9
	Side Bending 1

Foundational 2:
- Baseline Variation: Goal Instructions

Core:
- Building Variation 1: Increase Repetitions
  To build strength

Advanced:
- Challenge Variation 2: Increase Dynamics
  To introduce dynamic action to the Side Kick Series
- Challenge Variation 3: Lift Bottom Leg
  To prepare for the Single Leg Side Sit Up Series on the Ladder Barrel or Reformer.

The Order of Things
after Side Kicks - Up & Down

PERFORMANCE ORDER	EXERCISE	ADD NEXT #
1	Hundred	1
2	Roll Up	2
3	Single Leg Circle	3
4	Roll Like a Ball	4
5	Single Leg Pull Bent	5
6	Double Leg Pull Bent	6
7	Single Leg Pull Straight	9
8	Spine Stretch Forward	7
9	Introduction to Open Leg Rocker	17
10	Open Leg Rocker	18
11	Saw	15
12	Single Leg Kick Back	14
13	Introduction to Neck Pull	19
14	**SIDE KICKS - UP & DOWN**	**20**
15	Assisted Teaser 1	10
16	Assisted Teaser 2	11
17	Assisted Teaser 3*	12
18	Assisted Teaser 4*	13
19	Seal Without Beats	8
20	Introduction to the Push Up	16

*requires a spotter; omit if none

Side Kicks –
Front & Back

Add Next	21
Pages	163-165
Thread(s)	Stability 10
	Extension 2

Foundational 2:
- Baseline Variation: Goal Instructions
- Challenge Variation 1: Point and/or Flex
  To increase the stretch of the back of the leg and challenge coordination.

Advanced:
- Challenge Variation 2: Hold Kick of Leg
  To build strength in the depth of the stretch.
- Challenge Variation 3: Deepen Hold
  Teach this to prepare for the Big Splits on the Reformer or Mat.

Super Advanced:
- Challenge Variation 4: Old Fashioned
  Teach this before teaching the Star Old Fashioned or Snake on the Mat or Reformer.

The Order of Things
after Side Kicks - Front & Back

PERFORMANCE ORDER	EXERCISE	ADD NEXT #
1	Hundred	1
2	Roll Up	2
3	Single Leg Circle	3
4	Roll Like a Ball	4
5	Single Leg Pull Bent	5
6	Double Leg Pull Bent	6
7	Single Leg Pull Straight	9
8	Spine Stretch Forward	7
9	Introduction to Open Leg Rocker	17
10	Open Leg Rocker	18
11	Saw	15
12	Single Leg Kick Back	14
13	Introduction to Neck Pull	19
14	**SIDE KICKS - FRONT & BACK**	**21**
15	Side Kicks - Up & Down	20
16	Assisted Teaser 1	10
17	Assisted Teaser 2	11
18	Assisted Teaser 3*	12
19	Assisted Teaser 4*	13
20	Seal Without Beats	8
21	Introduction to the Push Up	16

*requires a spotter; omit if none

Side Kicks – Small Circles

Add Next	22
Pages	169-170
Thread(s)	Stability 11
	Extension 3
	Side Bending 2

Foundational 2:

- Building Variation 1: Increase Repetitions
  To build strength.
- Building Variation 2: Remove Pause in Circle When Heels Touch
  For the tense Student to increase understanding of fluid movement.
- Baseline Variation: Goal Instructions

Advanced:

- Challenge Variation 3: Increase Dynamics
  To introduce dynamic action to the Side Kick Series.
- Challenge Variation 4: Lift Bottom Leg
  To prepare for the Single Leg Side Sit Up Series.

This completes the Foundational Level sequence.

The Order of Things
after Side Kicks - Small Circles

PERFORMANCE ORDER	EXERCISE	ADD NEXT #
1	Hundred	1
2	Roll Up	2
3	Single Leg Circle	3
4	Roll Like a Ball	4
5	Single Leg Pull Bent	5
6	Double Leg Pull Bent	6
7	Single Leg Pull Straight	9
8	Spine Stretch Forward	7
9	Introduction to Open Leg Rocker	17
10	Open Leg Rocker	18
11	Saw	15
12	Single Leg Kick Back	14
13	Introduction to Neck Pull	19
14	Side Kicks - Front & Back	21
15	Side Kicks - Up & Down	20
16	**SIDE KICKS - SMALL CIRCLES**	**22**
17	Assisted Teaser 1	10
18	Assisted Teaser 2	11
19	Assisted Teaser 3*	12
20	Assisted Teaser 4*	13
21	Seal Without Beats	8
22	Introduction to the Push Up	16

*requires a spotter; omit if none

Single Leg Tick Tock

Add Next	23
Pages	51-52
Thread(s)	Twisting 2

No variations

Core:

- Baseline Variation: Goal Instructions

Advanced: Omit and replace with Single Leg Full Circle (Add Next #30).

Once Single Leg Tick Tock is added, it replaces the final two repetitions of the Single Leg Circle. The total number of repetitions of Single Leg Circle Flat and Single Leg Tick Tock, together, is five each way.

Performance Order Note: because we are now in the Core Level, Introduction to Open Leg Rocker is omitted from the Performance Order. But remember, these are guidelines only - the student may still require the stability preparation of Intro to Open Leg Rocker. But it will no longer be listed in the Performance Order charts.

The Order of Things
after Single Leg Tick Tock

PERFORMANCE ORDER	EXERCISE	ADD NEXT #
1	Hundred	1
2	Roll Up	2
3	Single Leg Circle	3
4	**SINGLE LEG TICK TOCK**	**23**
5	Roll Like a Ball	4
6	Single Leg Pull Bent	5
7	Double Leg Pull Bent	6
8	Single Leg Pull Straight	9
9	Spine Stretch Forward	7
10	Open Leg Rocker	18
11	Saw	15
12	Single Leg Kick Back	14
13	Introduction to Neck Pull	19
14	Side Kicks - Front & Back	21
15	Side Kicks - Up & Down	20
16	Side Kicks - Small Circles	22
17	Assisted Teaser 1	10
18	Assisted Teaser 2	11
19	Assisted Teaser 3*	12
20	Assisted Teaser 4*	13
21	Seal Without Beats	8
22	Introduction to the Push Up	16

*requires a spotter; omit if none

Double Leg Straight

Core:
- Building Variation 1: Hold the Thighs
  Great for hypermobile people and for people who don't use their entire stomach to support the Powerhouse.
- Building Variation 2: Lower to 45-Degrees
  For students who arch the back, lower legs too far, or lose control.
- Baseline Variation: Goal Instructions

Advanced:
- Challenge Variation 3: Single Leg Lower and Lift at 45-Degrees
  Great to balance a pelvis that rocks to one side when both legs lower.
- Challenge Variation 4: Double Leg Straight from 45-Degrees
  To build the movement of the last part of the Up Stretch on the Reformer.
- Challenge Variation 5: Pause at Bottom
  To build the last part of the Up Stretch on the Reformer.
- Challenge Variation 6: Beat as you Lower and Lift
- Challenge Variation 7: No Hands

Super Advanced:
- Challenge Variation 8: Beats at the Bottom
- Challenge Variation 9: Increase Counts
  Increases control, pelvic stability and abdominal strength. Teach before the Up Stretch on the Reformer.
- Challenge Variation 10: Hot Mat
  To increase dynamic action.

The Order of Things
after Double Leg Straight

PERFORMANCE ORDER	EXERCISE	ADD NEXT #
1	Hundred	1
2	Roll Up	2
3	Single Leg Circle	3
4	Single Leg Tick Tock	23
5	Roll Like a Ball	4
6	Single Leg Pull Bent	5
7	Double Leg Pull Bent	6
8	Single Leg Pull Straight	9
9	**DOUBLE LEG STRAIGHT**	**24**
10	Spine Stretch Forward	7
11	Open Leg Rocker	18
12	Saw	15
13	Single Leg Kick Back	14
14	Introduction to Neck Pull	19
15	Side Kicks - Front & Back	21
16	Side Kicks - Up & Down	20
17	Side Kicks - Small Circles	22
18	Assisted Teaser 1	10
19	Assisted Teaser 2	11
20	Assisted Teaser 3*	12
21	Assisted Teaser 4*	13
22	Seal Without Beats	8
23	Introduction to the Push Up	16

*requires a spotter; omit if none

Criss Cross

Add Next	25
Pages	77-82
Thread(s)	Twisting 3

Core:

- Building Variation 1: Introduction to Criss Cross
  To create a strong foundation and pelvic stability.
  - Step 1: feet down
  - Step 2: knee float
  - Step 3: extend opposite leg
- Building Variation 2: Change with Knees into Chest
  To focus on the lift of the upper body and use the upper abdominals.
- Baseline Variation: Goal Instructions
- Challenge Variation 3: Change in Hidden Teaser
  To deepen the work of the lower abdominals.

Advanced:

- Challenge Variation 5: Extended Leg Pause
  To challenge both upper and lower abdominals.
- Challenge Variation 6: Execute with Straight Legs
  To add stretch and strength for the back of the legs.

Super Advanced:

- Challenge Variation 7: Rolling Up into Teaser
  To increase the connection to functional movement when twisting.
- Challenge Variation 8: Fish
  To strengthen the side body.
  - Optional Breakdown: 2 sets only lift legs, 2 sets only lift upper body, final 2 sets full Fish
- Challenge Variation 9: River Roll
  Use this variation for the student who likes to shorten or add side bending to rotation.
- Challenge Variation 10: Reverse Twist
  For the student who adds side bending or shortens one side on Criss Cross.
- Challenge Variation 11: Hip Lift/Bent Knee at 90-Degrees or Straight Line
  For the student who has trouble lifting the hip on the Side Bend.

Performance Order Note: Challenge Variation 11 may be placed after Mermaid as an introduction to Side Bend or during the Side Kick Series before transition to the other side.

The Order of Things
after Criss Cross

PERFORMANCE ORDER	EXERCISE	ADD NEXT #
1	Hundred	1
2	Roll Up	2
3	Single Leg Circle	3
4	Single Leg Tick Tock	23
5	Roll Like a Ball	4
6	Single Leg Pull Bent	5
7	Double Leg Pull Bent	6
8	Single Leg Pull Straight	9
9	Double Leg Straight	24
10	**CRISS CROSS**	**25**
11	Spine Stretch Forward	7
12	Open Leg Rocker	18
13	Saw	15
14	Single Leg Kick Back	14
15	Introduction to Neck Pull	19
16	Side Kicks - Front & Back	21
17	Side Kicks - Up & Down	20
18	Side Kicks - Small Circles	22
19	Assisted Teaser 1	10
20	Assisted Teaser 2	11
21	Assisted Teaser 3*	12
22	Assisted Teaser 4*	13
23	Seal Without Beats	8
24	Introduction to the Push Up	16

*requires a spotter; omit if none

Corkscrew Flat

Add Next	26
Pages	97-100
Thread(s)	Twisting 4

Core:

- Building Variation 1: Sign of the Cross – Flat Back
  To establish a strong center and connects movement of legs to Powerhouse.
- Building Variation 2: Open Leg Tick Tock
  To Introduce the rotation of the pelvis against a stable upper back.
- Building Variation 3: Open Leg Tick Tock 2
  From the Teaching notes - teach this in preparation for Corkscrew Tail Off.
- Building Variation 4: Little Tick Tock
  To introduce rotating the pelvis with the weight of two legs against a stable upper back.
- Baseline Variation: Goal Instructions

The Order of Things after Corkscrew Flat

PERFORMANCE ORDER	EXERCISE	ADD NEXT #
1	Hundred	1
2	Roll Up	2
3	Single Leg Circle	3
4	Single Leg Tick Tock	23
5	Roll Like a Ball	4
6	Single Leg Pull Bent	5
7	Double Leg Pull Bent	6
8	Single Leg Pull Straight	9
9	Double Leg Straight	24
10	Criss Cross	25
11	Spine Stretch Forward	7
12	Open Leg Rocker	18
13	**CORKSCREW FLAT**	**26**
14	Saw	15
15	Single Leg Kick Back	14
16	Introduction to Neck Pull	19
17	Side Kicks - Front & Back	21
18	Side Kicks - Up & Down	20
19	Side Kicks - Small Circles	22
20	Assisted Teaser 1	10
21	Assisted Teaser 2	11
22	Assisted Teaser 3*	12
23	Assisted Teaser 4*	13
24	Seal Without Beats	8
25	Introduction to the Push Up	16

*requires a spotter; omit if none

Neck Roll

Add Next	27
Pages	113-114
Thread(s)	Twisting 5
	Extension 3

No variations

Core:

- Baseline Variation: Goal Instructions

The Order of Things
after Neck Roll

PERFORMANCE ORDER	EXERCISE	ADD NEXT #
1	Hundred	1
2	Roll Up	2
3	Single Leg Circle	3
4	Single Leg Tick Tock	23
5	Roll Like a Ball	4
6	Single Leg Pull Bent	5
7	Double Leg Pull Bent	6
8	Single Leg Pull Straight	9
9	Double Leg Straight	24
10	Criss Cross	25
11	Spine Stretch Forward	7
12	Open Leg Rocker	18
13	Corkscrew Flat	26
14	Saw	15
15	**NECK ROLL**	**27**
16	Single Leg Kick Back	14
17	Introduction to Neck Pull	19
18	Side Kicks - Front & Back	21
19	Side Kicks - Up & Down	20
20	Side Kicks - Small Circles	22
21	Assisted Teaser 1	10
22	Assisted Teaser 2	11
23	Assisted Teaser 3*	12
24	Assisted Teaser 4*	13
25	Seal Without Beats	8
26	Introduction to the Push Up	16

*requires a spotter; omit if none

Teaser 1

No Building Variations. The Building Variations for Teaser 1 are the prior exercises of the Articulation Thread. If the student isn't ready, do not Pass Go, do not Collect $200.

Core:
- Baseline Variation: Goal Instructions

Advanced:
- Challenge Variation 1: Seated Teaser
  Teach in preparation for introducing Jackknife and Boomerang
- Challenge Variation 2: Half Way Down
  To develop Powerhouse and strength.

Super Advanced:
- Challenge Variation 3: Arms to Ears
  To challenge Powerhouse.

Performance Order Note: when Teaser 1 is added, the Assisted Teaser variations are omitted from the Performance Order. But again, these are guidelines not rules, you/your student may need a Teaser Prep before executing Teaser 1. However, the Assisted Teasers will no longer appear in the Performance Order.

The Order of Things
after Teaser 1

PERFORMANCE ORDER	EXERCISE	ADD NEXT #
1	Hundred	1
2	Roll Up	2
3	Single Leg Circle	3
4	Single Leg Tick Tock	23
5	Roll Like a Ball	4
6	Single Leg Pull Bent	5
7	Double Leg Pull Bent	6
8	Single Leg Pull Straight	9
9	Double Leg Straight	24
10	Criss Cross	25
11	Spine Stretch Forward	7
12	Open Leg Rocker	18
13	Corkscrew Flat	26
14	Saw	15
15	Neck Roll	27
16	Single Leg Kick Back	14
17	Introduction to Neck Pull	19
18	Side Kicks - Front & Back	21
19	Side Kicks - Up & Down	20
20	Side Kicks - Small Circles	22
21	**TEASER 1**	**28**
22	Seal Without Beats	8
23	Introduction to the Push Up	16

Double Leg Kick Back

Add Next	29
Pages	125-128
Thread(s)	Stability 13
	Extension 4

Core:

- Building Variation 1: Single Leg Stretch
- Baseline Variation: Goal Instructions
- Challenge Variation 2: Clasped Hands on Buttocks
  To open the front of the shoulder
- Challenge Variation 3: Clasped Hands Lifted
  To open and stretch the shoulders and across the collarbones.
- Challenge Variation 4: Flat Hands Palms Face Up
  To stretch the triceps and open the chest.
- Challenge Variation 5: Finger Tip Elbow
  To stretch arms, shoulders and chest.
- Challenge Variation 6: Reverse Prayer Palms Up
  For the deepest stretch of the front body.

Super Advanced:

- Challenge Variation 7: Lift Legs Off Mat
  Introduce this prior to Swan Dive (Add Next #68)

The Order of Things
after Double Leg Kick Back

PERFORMANCE ORDER	EXERCISE	ADD NEXT #
1	Hundred	1
2	Roll Up	2
3	Single Leg Circle	3
4	Single Leg Tick Tock	23
5	Roll Like a Ball	4
6	Single Leg Pull Bent	5
7	Double Leg Pull Bent	6
8	Single Leg Pull Straight	9
9	Double Leg Straight	24
10	Criss Cross	25
11	Spine Stretch Forward	7
12	Open Leg Rocker	18
13	Corkscrew Flat	26
14	Saw	15
15	Neck Roll	27
16	Single Leg Kick Back	14
17	**DOUBLE LEG KICK BACK**	**29**
18	Introduction to Neck Pull	19
19	Side Kicks - Front & Back	21
20	Side Kicks - Up & Down	20
21	Side Kicks - Small Circles	22
22	Teaser 1	28
23	Seal Without Beats	8
24	Introduction to the Push Up	16

Single Leg Circle Full

Core:

- Baseline Variation: Goal Instructions

Super Advanced:

- Challenge Variation 1: Lift Bottom Leg

As with the Single Leg Tick Tock the total number of repetitions of Single Leg Circle plus Single Leg Circle Full is five each way, not five of each.

Performance Order Note: when Single Leg Circle Full is added, Single Leg Tick Tock is omitted. The twisting preparation of the Single Leg Tick Tock is now replaced with a larger expression of the twisting action with Single Leg Circle Full. Again, these are guidelines, not rules. You may wish to leave the preparatory Tick Tock in your/your client's routine, but it will no longer appear in the Performance Order chart.

The Order of Things
after Single Leg Circle Full

PERFORMANCE ORDER	EXERCISE	ADD NEXT #
1	Hundred	1
2	Roll Up	2
3	Single Leg Circle	3
4	**SINGLE LEG CIRCLE FULL**	**30**
5	Roll Like a Ball	4
6	Single Leg Pull Bent	5
7	Double Leg Pull Bent	6
8	Single Leg Pull Straight	9
9	Double Leg Straight	24
10	Criss Cross	25
11	Spine Stretch Forward	7
12	Open Leg Rocker	18
13	Corkscrew Flat	26
14	Saw	15
15	Neck Roll	27
16	Single Leg Kick Back	14
17	Double Leg Kick Back	29
18	Introduction to Neck Pull	19
19	Side Kicks - Front & Back	21
20	Side Kicks - Up & Down	20
21	Side Kicks - Small Circles	22
22	Teaser 1	28
23	Seal Without Beats	8
24	Introduction to the Push Up	16

The Neck Pull

Add Next	31
Pages	135-139
Thread(s)	Articulation 9

Core:

- Building Variation 1: Two Up One Down
  For the student who skips vertebrae when rolling up or down.
- Building Variation 2: Elbows In
  For tight shoulders and upper back.
- Building Variation 3: Pause
  To clarify articulation through the spine and build abdominal control.
- Building Variation 4: No Pulse
  To create smooth flow.
- Baseline Variation: Goal Instructions

Advanced:

- Challenge Variation 5: Flat Back
  To develop Long Spinal Massage on the Reformer.

Performance Order Note: once The Neck Pull is added, it replaces Intro to Neck Pull in the Performance Order.

The Order of Things
after The Neck Pull

PERFORMANCE ORDER	EXERCISE	ADD NEXT #
1	Hundred	1
2	Roll Up	2
3	Single Leg Circle	3
4	Single Leg Circle Full	30
5	Roll Like a Ball	4
6	Single Leg Pull Bent	5
7	Double Leg Pull Bent	6
8	Single Leg Pull Straight	9
9	Double Leg Straight	24
10	Criss Cross	25
11	Spine Stretch Forward	7
12	Open Leg Rocker	18
13	Corkscrew Flat	26
14	Saw	15
15	Neck Roll	27
16	Single Leg Kick Back	14
17	Double Leg Kick Back	29
18	**THE NECK PULL**	**31**
19	Side Kicks - Front & Back	21
20	Side Kicks - Up & Down	20
21	Side Kicks - Small Circles	22
22	Teaser 1	28
23	Seal Without Beats	8
24	Introduction to the Push Up	16

Corkscrew Tail Off

Add Next	32
Pages	101-102
Thread(s)	Twisting 7

Core:
- Building Variation 1: Sign of the Cross – Hip Lift
  To introduce the points that the pelvis will hit during the twist of the Corkscrew.
- Baseline Variation: Goal Instructions

The Order of Things
after Corkscrew Tail Off

PERFORMANCE ORDER	EXERCISE	ADD NEXT #
1	Hundred	1
2	Roll Up	2
3	Single Leg Circle	3
4	Single Leg Circle Full	30
5	Roll Like a Ball	4
6	Single Leg Pull Bent	5
7	Double Leg Pull Bent	6
8	Single Leg Pull Straight	9
9	Double Leg Straight	24
10	Criss Cross	25
11	Spine Stretch Forward	7
12	Open Leg Rocker	18
13	Corkscrew Flat	26
14	**CORKSCREW TAIL OFF**	**32**
15	Saw	15
16	Neck Roll	27
17	Single Leg Kick Back	14
18	Double Leg Kick Back	29
19	The Neck Pull	31
20	Side Kicks - Front & Back	21
21	Side Kicks - Up & Down	20
22	Side Kicks - Small Circles	22
23	Teaser 1	28
24	Seal Without Beats	8
25	Introduction to the Push Up	16

Side Kicks - Bicycle

Add Next	33
Pages	189-191
Thread(s)	Stability 14
	Extension 6

Core:

- Baseline Variation: Goal Instructions
  Note: see Side Kicks Setup and Focus, pages 159-162 for teaching tips and arm position options

Advanced:

- Challenge Variation 1: Pause
  Note: Arm Position is both hands behind the head

Super Advanced:

- Challenge Variation 2: Hold & Stretch

The Order of Things
after Side Kicks - Bicycle

PERFORMANCE ORDER	EXERCISE	ADD NEXT #
1	Hundred	1
2	Roll Up	2
3	Single Leg Circle	3
4	Single Leg Circle Full	30
5	Roll Like a Ball	4
6	Single Leg Pull Bent	5
7	Double Leg Pull Bent	6
8	Single Leg Pull Straight	9
9	Double Leg Straight	24
10	Criss Cross	25
11	Spine Stretch Forward	7
12	Open Leg Rocker	18
13	Corkscrew Flat	26
14	Corkscrew Tail Off	32
15	Saw	15
16	Neck Roll	27
17	Single Leg Kick Back	14
18	Double Leg Kick Back	29
19	The Neck Pull	31
20	Side Kicks - Front & Back	21
21	Side Kicks - Up & Down	20
22	Side Kicks - Small Circles	22
23	**SIDE KICKS - BICYCLE**	**33**
24	Teaser 1	28
25	Seal Without Beats	8
26	Introduction to the Push Up	16

Seal With Beats

Add Next	34
Pages	273-274
Thread(s)	Rolling (Forward) 4

Core:
- Baseline Variation: Goal Instructions

Advanced:
- Challenge Variation 1: Inch Balance
- Challenge Variation 2: Extended Seal

Performance Order Note: Once Seal With Beats is added to the workout, it replaces Seal Without Beats in the Performance Order.

**The Order of Things
after Seal with Beats**

PERFORMANCE ORDER	EXERCISE	ADD NEXT #
1	Hundred	1
2	Roll Up	2
3	Single Leg Circle	3
4	Single Leg Circle Full	30
5	Roll Like a Ball	4
6	Single Leg Pull Bent	5
7	Double Leg Pull Bent	6
8	Single Leg Pull Straight	9
9	Double Leg Straight	24
10	Criss Cross	25
11	Spine Stretch Forward	7
12	Open Leg Rocker	18
13	Corkscrew Flat	26
14	Corkscrew Tail Off	32
15	Saw	15
16	Neck Roll	27
17	Single Leg Kick Back	14
18	Double Leg Kick Back	29
19	The Neck Pull	31
20	Side Kicks - Front & Back	21
21	Side Kicks - Up & Down	20
22	Side Kicks - Small Circles	22
23	Side Kicks - Bicycle	33
24	Teaser 1	28
25	**SEAL WITH BEATS**	**34**
26	Introduction to the Push Up	16

Can Can

Add Next	35
Pages	227-228
Thread(s)	Twisting 9

Core:

- Building Variation 1: Simple Can Can
  To focus and isolate rotation.
- Building Variation 2: Can Can Elbows to Mat
  For very tight shoulders or hand and wrist issues.
- Baseline Variation: Goal Instructions
- Challenge Variation 3: Reverse Can Can

Advanced +: replace with Hip Circles (*Add Next #56*)

The Order of Things
after Can Can

PERFORMANCE ORDER	EXERCISE	ADD NEXT #
1	Hundred	1
2	Roll Up	2
3	Single Leg Circle	3
4	Single Leg Circle Full	30
5	Roll Like a Ball	4
6	Single Leg Pull Bent	5
7	Double Leg Pull Bent	6
8	Single Leg Pull Straight	9
9	Double Leg Straight	24
10	Criss Cross	25
11	Spine Stretch Forward	7
12	Open Leg Rocker	18
13	Corkscrew Flat	26
14	Corkscrew Tail Off	32
15	Saw	15
16	Neck Roll	27
17	Single Leg Kick Back	14
18	Double Leg Kick Back	29
19	The Neck Pull	31
20	Side Kicks - Front & Back	21
21	Side Kicks - Up & Down	20
22	Side Kicks - Small Circles	22
23	Side Kicks - Bicycle	33
24	Teaser 1	28
25	**CAN CAN**	**35**
26	Seal With Beats	34
27	Introduction to the Push Up	16

Pilates Push Up

Add Next	36
Pages	285-289
Thread(s)	Stabilization 15 [Articulation]

Core:
- Baseline Variation: Goal Instructions

Advanced:
- Challenge Variation 1: Increase Repetitions
- Challenge Variation 2: Heels Up
  To build balance and control.
- Challenge Variation 3: One Leg
  Note: teach after Leg Pull Front (Add Next #57)

Super Advanced:
- Challenge Variation 4: One Leg – Heels Up
  Note: teach after Leg Pull Front (Add Next #57)
- Challenge Variation 5: Clap Hands
  To dynamically connect upper body.
- Challenge Variation 6: Clap Legs
  To dynamically connect lower body.
- Challenge Variation 7: Clap Hands & Legs
  To dynamically connect whole body.
- Challenge Variation 8: One Arm
  To build cross body stability.
- Challenge Variation 9: One Arm/One Leg Hold
  To challenge balance an control.
- Challenge Variation 10: Wide Arms
  To work the chest and improve Rowing Series on Reformer.
- Challenge Variation 11: Wide Arms & Legs
  To develop the Up Stretch Combination on the Reformer and the Squirrel on the Cadillac.
- Challenge Variation 12: Head Press
  To prepare for Head Stands on the Reformer

Performance Order Note: The Intro to the Push Up is a breakdown of the Push Up, taking out the elbow bend (you know, the actual pushing up part of the Push Up). So once the full Push Up is added, it replaces Intro to Push Up in the Performance Order.

The Order of Things
after Pilates Push Up

PERFORMANCE ORDER	EXERCISE	ADD NEXT #
1	Hundred	1
2	Roll Up	2
3	Single Leg Circle	3
4	Single Leg Circle Full	30
5	Roll Like a Ball	4
6	Single Leg Pull Bent	5
7	Double Leg Pull Bent	6
8	Single Leg Pull Straight	9
9	Double Leg Straight	24
10	Criss Cross	25
11	Spine Stretch Forward	7
12	Open Leg Rocker	18
13	Corkscrew Flat	26
14	Corkscrew Tail Off	32
15	Saw	15
16	Neck Roll	27
17	Single Leg Kick Back	14
18	Double Leg Kick Back	29
19	The Neck Pull	31
20	Side Kicks - Front & Back	21
21	Side Kicks - Up & Down	20
22	Side Kicks - Small Circles	22
23	Side Kicks - Bicycle	33
24	Teaser 1	28
25	Can Can	35
26	Seal With Beats	34
27	**PILATES PUSH UP**	**36**

Side Kicks – Medium Circles

Add Next	37
Pages	171-172
Thread(s)	Stability 16
	Extension 7
	Side Bending 3

Core:

- Building Variation 1: Increase Repetitions
  To build strength.
- Building Variation 2: Remove Pause in Circle When Heels Touch
  For the tense student to increase understanding of fluid movement.
- Baseline Variation: Goal Instructions

Advanced:

- Challenge Variation 3: Increase Dynamics
  To introduce dynamic action to the Side Kick Series.
- Challenge Variation 4: Lift Bottom Leg
  To prepare for the Single Leg Side Sit Up Series on the apparatus.

From Side Kicks Set Up & Focus (page 159-60): "When working the Side Kick Series, classically Front & Back, Up & Down, Small Circles, Bicycle, and Large Circles are executed. The other variations are added as per need of the Student." This variation of Side Kick is, therefore, optional. Use this variation to challenge Side Kicks - Small Circles.

70

The Order of Things
after Side Kicks – Medium Circles

PERFORMANCE ORDER	EXERCISE	ADD NEXT #
1	Hundred	1
2	Roll Up	2
3	Single Leg Circle	3
4	Single Leg Circle Full	30
5	Roll Like a Ball	4
6	Single Leg Pull Bent	5
7	Double Leg Pull Bent	6
8	Single Leg Pull Straight	9
9	Double Leg Straight	24
10	Criss Cross	25
11	Spine Stretch Forward	7
12	Open Leg Rocker	18
13	Corkscrew Flat	26
14	Corkscrew Tail Off	32
15	Saw	15
16	Neck Roll	27
17	Single Leg Kick Back	14
18	Double Leg Kick Back	29
19	The Neck Pull	31
20	Side Kicks - Front & Back	21
21	Side Kicks - Up & Down	20
22	Side Kicks - Small Circles	22
23	**SIDE KICKS - MEDIUM CIRCLES***	**37**
24	Side Kicks - Bicycle	33
25	Teaser 1	28
26	Can Can	35
27	Seal With Beats	34
28	Pilates Push Up	36

*optional if needed by student

Swan Preparation

Add Next	38
Pages	115-118
Thread(s)	Stability 17
	Extension 8

Core:

- Building Variation 1: Upper Back Prep
  To prepare tight shoulders and the upper back.
- Building Variation 2: Upper Back Prep 2
  To prepare tight shoulders and upper backs.
- Building Variation 3: Push Up Swan
  To Introduce the lift and upper body position for the Swan.
- Baseline Variation: Goal Instructions
- Challenge Variation 4: Alternating Upper Body and Lower Body Lift
  For students who like to throw the arms and legs and use the lower back. Aids in teaching control.
- Challenge Variation 5: Hands Behind the Head
  For the student who closes the chest on the rock forward, and for tight shoulders.

Advanced +: replace with Swan Dive (*Add Next #68*)

The Order of Things
after Swan Preparation

PERFORMANCE ORDER	EXERCISE	ADD NEXT #
1	Hundred	1
2	Roll Up	2
3	Single Leg Circle	3
4	Single Leg Circle Full	30
5	Roll Like a Ball	4
6	Single Leg Pull Bent	5
7	Double Leg Pull Bent	6
8	Single Leg Pull Straight	9
9	Double Leg Straight	24
10	Criss Cross	25
11	Spine Stretch Forward	7
12	Open Leg Rocker	18
13	Corkscrew Flat	26
14	Corkscrew Tail Off	32
15	Saw	15
16	Neck Roll	27
17	**SWAN PREPARATION**	**38**
18	Single Leg Kick Back	14
19	Double Leg Kick Back	29
20	The Neck Pull	31
21	Side Kicks - Front & Back	21
22	Side Kicks - Up & Down	20
23	Side Kicks - Small Circles	22
24	Side Kicks - Medium Circles*	37
25	Side Kicks - Bicycle	33
26	Teaser 1	28
27	Can Can	35
28	Seal With Beats	34
29	Pilates Push Up	36

*optional if needed by student

Mermaid

Add Next	39
Pages	253-256
Thread(s)	Side Bending 3

Core 2:

- Building Variation 1: Bent Arm Slide
  To build stability of side body.
- Building Variation 2: Straight Arm Half Slide
  To continue to build stability of side body with a long spine and correct shoulder engagement.
- Baseline Variation: Goal Instructions

Advanced:

- Challenge Variation 3: Bent Arm Wrap
  To increase stretch.
- Challenge Variation 4: Bent Arm Wrap with Head Turn
  To increase stretch and introduce a twist to the side bend, as in Snake & Twist.

Super Advanced:

- Challenge Variation 5: Bent Arm Wrap with Twist
  To increase stretch and introduce a twist to the side bend, as in Snake & Twist
- Challenge Variation 6: Hip Lift
  To build the side body strength for Side Bend.

The Order of Things
after Mermaid

PERFORMANCE ORDER	EXERCISE	ADD NEXT #
1	Hundred	1
2	Roll Up	2
3	Single Leg Circle	3
4	Single Leg Circle Full	30
5	Roll Like a Ball	4
6	Single Leg Pull Bent	5
7	Double Leg Pull Bent	6
8	Single Leg Pull Straight	9
9	Double Leg Straight	24
10	Criss Cross	25
11	Spine Stretch Forward	7
12	Open Leg Rocker	18
13	Corkscrew Flat	26
14	Corkscrew Tail Off	32
15	Saw	15
16	Neck Roll	27
17	Swan Preparation	38
18	Single Leg Kick Back	14
19	Double Leg Kick Back	29
20	The Neck Pull	31
21	Side Kicks - Front & Back	21
22	Side Kicks - Up & Down	20
23	Side Kicks - Small Circles	22
24	Side Kicks - Medium Circles*	37
25	Side Kicks - Bicycle	33
26	Teaser 1	28
27	Can Can	35
28	**MERMAID**	**39**
29	Seal With Beats	34
30	Pilates Push Up	36

*optional if needed by student

Spine Twist

Add Next	40
Pages	151-154
Thread(s)	Twisting 9

Core 2:

- Unofficial Building Variation from Teaching section: Feet pressed against a wall
  If the heels shift as they twist.
- Building Variation 1: Hands on Shoulders
  For the student who twists with, or drops, their arms
- Building Variation 2: Clasped Hands – Flat Hands
  If the arms go behind the side body when they twist.
- Building Variation 3: Fingertip to Elbow
  For the student who needs to lift up out of the waist and flares the ribs.
- Building Variation 4: Hand to Shoulder – Elbows Down
  For shoulder issues and student who arch the upper back while twisting.
- Baseline Variation: Goal Instructions

Advanced:

- Challenge Variation 5: Prayer Hands
  For the Advanced Student who lifts their shoulders when they twist and needs to open their chest.
- Challenge Variation 6: One Arm Up - One Arm Down
  For scoliosis and people who sink onto one side.
- Challenge Variation 7: Pole Looped Over
  For stiff people to help keep the back and shoulders open and to prevent arms from going behind the shoulders.
- Challenge Variation 8: Pole Looped Under – Ribs On & Ribs Off
  For people who round their shoulders forward and prevent the arms from going behind the shoulder.

Super Advanced:

- Challenge Variation 9: Pulse
  To increase the twist.
- Challenge Variation 10: Head Turn
  To increase full rotation. Great to teach before Short Box Off Hip on the Reformer.
- Challenge Variation 11: Wide Arms
  Opens the chest.

- Challenge Variation 12: Reversed Breathing
To challenge the breath and coordination. For students who don't fully exhale.

The Order of Things
after Spine Twist

PERFORMANCE ORDER	EXERCISE	ADD NEXT #
1	Hundred	1
2	Roll Up	2
3	Single Leg Circle	3
4	Single Leg Circle Full	30
5	Roll Like a Ball	4
6	Single Leg Pull Bent	5
7	Double Leg Pull Bent	6
8	Single Leg Pull Straight	9
9	Double Leg Straight	24
10	Criss Cross	25
11	Spine Stretch Forward	7
12	Open Leg Rocker	18
13	Corkscrew Flat	26
14	Corkscrew Tail Off	32
15	Saw	15
16	Neck Roll	27
17	Swan Preparation	38
18	Single Leg Kick Back	14
19	Double Leg Kick Back	29
20	The Neck Pull	31
21	**SPINE TWIST**	**40**
22	Side Kicks - Front & Back	21
23	Side Kicks - Up & Down	20
24	Side Kicks - Small Circles	22
25	Side Kicks - Medium Circles*	37
26	Side Kicks - Bicycle	33
27	Teaser 1	28
28	Can Can	35
29	Mermaid	39
30	Seal With Beats	34
31	Pilates Push Up	36

*optional if needed by student

Teaser 2

Core 2:

- Baseline Variation: Goal Instructions

Advanced:

- Challenge Variation 1: Arms to Ears
  Teach before Up Stretch on the Reformer.

Super Advanced:

- Challenge Variation 2: Circles in Opposition
  Teach after Hips Circles (on the Mat) and before Snake & Twist on the Reformer.

The Order of Things
after Teaser 2

PERFORMANCE ORDER	EXERCISE	ADD NEXT #
1	Hundred	1
2	Roll Up	2
3	Single Leg Circle	3
4	Single Leg Circle Full	30
5	Roll Like a Ball	4
6	Single Leg Pull Bent	5
7	Double Leg Pull Bent	6
8	Single Leg Pull Straight	9
9	Double Leg Straight	24
10	Criss Cross	25
11	Spine Stretch Forward	7
12	Open Leg Rocker	18
13	Corkscrew Flat	26
14	Corkscrew Tail Off	32
15	Saw	15
16	Neck Roll	27
17	Swan Preparation	38
18	Single Leg Kick Back	14
19	Double Leg Kick Back	29
20	The Neck Pull	31
21	Spine Twist	40
22	Side Kicks - Front & Back	21
23	Side Kicks - Up & Down	20
24	Side Kicks - Small Circles	22
25	Side Kicks - Medium Circles*	37
26	Side Kicks - Bicycle	33
27	Teaser 1	28
28	**TEASER 2**	**41**
29	Can Can	35
30	Mermaid	39
31	Seal With Beats	34
32	Pilates Push Up	36

*optional if needed by student

Side Kicks -
Inner Thigh Lifts

Add Next	42
Pages	175-176
Thread(s)	Stability 19

Core 2:
- Building Variation 1: Increase Repetitions
  To build strength.
- Building Variation 2: Quick Lower & Lift
  To teach rapid muscle firing needed for dynamic action of Advanced exercises.
- Baseline Variation: Goal Instructions

Advanced:
- Challenge Variation 3: Increase Dynamics
  To increase dynamic action in the Side Kick Series

Super Advanced:
- Challenge Variation 4: Add Hold on Lift
  To increase inner thigh strength.

Note: Inner Thigh Lifts is one of the optional Side Kicks, added only if the student needs additional inner thigh work.

The Order of Things
after Side Kicks – Inner Thigh Lifts

PERFORMANCE ORDER	EXERCISE	ADD NEXT #
1	Hundred	1
2	Roll Up	2
3	Single Leg Circle	3
4	Single Leg Circle Full	30
5	Roll Like a Ball	4
6	Single Leg Pull Bent	5
7	Double Leg Pull Bent	6
8	Single Leg Pull Straight	9
9	Double Leg Straight	24
10	Criss Cross	25
11	Spine Stretch Forward	7
12	Open Leg Rocker	18
13	Corkscrew Flat	26
14	Corkscrew Tail Off	32
15	Saw	15
16	Neck Roll	27
17	Swan Preparation	38
18	Single Leg Kick Back	14
19	Double Leg Kick Back	29
20	The Neck Pull	31
21	Spine Twist	40
22	Side Kicks - Front & Back	21
23	Side Kicks - Up & Down	20
24	Side Kicks - Small Circles	22
25	Side Kicks - Medium Circles*	37
26	**SIDE KICKS - INNER THIGH LIFTS***	**42**
27	Side Kicks - Bicycle	33
28	Teaser 1	28
29	Teaser 2	41
30	Can Can	35
31	Mermaid	39
32	Seal With Beats	34
33	Pilates Push Up	36

*optional if needed by student

Side Kicks – Inner Thigh Circles

Add Next	43
Pages	177-178
Thread(s)	Stability 20

Core 2:

- Building Variation 1: Increase Repetitions
  Use to build strength.
- Building Variation 2: Quick Circles
  Use to teach rapid muscle firing needed for dynamic action of advanced exercises.
- Baseline Variation: Goal Instructions

Advanced:

- Challenge Variation 3: Increase Dynamics
  To increase dynamic action in the Side Kick Series.

Super Advanced:

- Challenge Variation 4: Add Hold on Lift
  To increase inner thigh strength.

Note: Inner Thigh Circles is one of the optional Side Kicks, added only if the student needs additional inner thigh work.

The Order of Things
after Side Kicks – Inner Thigh Circles

PERFORMANCE ORDER	EXERCISE	ADD NEXT #
1	Hundred	1
2	Roll Up	2
3	Single Leg Circle	3
4	Single Leg Circle Full	30
5	Roll Like a Ball	4
6	Single Leg Pull Bent	5
7	Double Leg Pull Bent	6
8	Single Leg Pull Straight	9
9	Double Leg Straight	24
10	Criss Cross	25
11	Spine Stretch Forward	7
12	Open Leg Rocker	18
13	Corkscrew Flat	26
14	Corkscrew Tail Off	32
15	Saw	15
16	Neck Roll	27
17	Swan Preparation	38
18	Single Leg Kick Back	14
19	Double Leg Kick Back	29
20	The Neck Pull	31
21	Spine Twist	40
22	Side Kicks - Front & Back	21
23	Side Kicks - Up & Down	20
24	Side Kicks - Small Circles	22
25	Side Kicks - Medium Circles*	37
26	Side Kicks - Inner Thigh Lifts*	42
27	**SIDE KICKS - INNER THIGH CIRCLES***	**43**
28	Side Kicks - Bicycle	33
29	Teaser 1	28
30	Teaser 2	41
31	Can Can	35
32	Mermaid	39
33	Seal With Beats	34
34	Pilates Push Up	36

*optional if needed by student

Side Kicks - Side Bicycle

Add Next	44
Pages	179-181
Thread(s)	Stability 21 Side Bending 5

Core 2:

- Baseline Variation: Goal Instructions

Advanced:

- Challenge Variation 1: Both Hands Behind the Head
  Use to challenge balance.

Super Advanced:

- Challenge Variation 2: Hold & Stretch

Note: Side Bicycle is one of the optional Side Kicks, added only if needed.

The Order of Things
after Side Kicks – Side Bicycle

PERFORMANCE ORDER	EXERCISE	ADD NEXT #
1	Hundred	1
2	Roll Up	2
3	Single Leg Circle	3
4	Single Leg Circle Full	30
5	Roll Like a Ball	4
6	Single Leg Pull Bent	5
7	Double Leg Pull Bent	6
8	Single Leg Pull Straight	9
9	Double Leg Straight	24
10	Criss Cross	25
11	Spine Stretch Forward	7
12	Open Leg Rocker	18
13	Corkscrew Flat	26
14	Corkscrew Tail Off	32
15	Saw	15
16	Neck Roll	27
17	Swan Preparation	38
18	Single Leg Kick Back	14
19	Double Leg Kick Back	29
20	The Neck Pull	31
21	Spine Twist	40
22	Side Kicks - Front & Back	21
23	Side Kicks - Up & Down	20
24	Side Kicks - Small Circles	22
25	Side Kicks - Medium Circles*	37
26	Side Kicks - Inner Thigh Lifts*	42
27	Side Kicks - Inner Thigh Circles*	43
28	**SIDE KICKS - SIDE BICYCLE***	**44**
29	Side Kicks - Bicycle	33
30	Teaser 1	28
31	Teaser 2	41
32	Can Can	35
33	Mermaid	39
34	Seal With Beats	34
35	Pilates Push Up	36

*optional if needed by student

Side Kicks -
Double Leg Lifts

Add Next	45
Pages	183-184
Thread(s)	Stability 22 Side Bending 6

Core 2:
- Baseline Variation: Goal Instructions

Advanced:
- Challenge Variation 1: Upper Body Lift
  To develop the side bend strength needed for Kneeling Side Kicks and the Side Bend.

Super Advanced:
- Challenge Variation 2: Fish
  To develop the side bend strength needed for Kneeling Side Kicks and the Side Bend.

Note: Double Leg Lifts is one of the optional Side Kicks that is added only if the student needs it. One purpose noted in Side Kicks Series Set up and Focus is *for love handles.*

The Order of Things
after Side Kicks - Double Leg Lifts

PERFORMANCE ORDER	EXERCISE	ADD NEXT #
1	Hundred	1
2	Roll Up	2
3	Single Leg Circle	3
4	Single Leg Circle Full	30
5	Roll Like a Ball	4
6	Single Leg Pull Bent	5
7	Double Leg Pull Bent	6
8	Single Leg Pull Straight	9
9	Double Leg Straight	24
10	Criss Cross	25
11	Spine Stretch Forward	7
12	Open Leg Rocker	18
13	Corkscrew Flat	26
14	Corkscrew Tail Off	32
15	Saw	15
16	Neck Roll	27
17	Swan Preparation	38
18	Single Leg Kick Back	14
19	Double Leg Kick Back	29
20	The Neck Pull	31
21	Spine Twist	40
22	Side Kicks - Front & Back	21
23	Side Kicks - Up & Down	20
24	Side Kicks - Small Circles	22
25	Side Kicks - Medium Circles*	37
26	Side Kicks - Inner Thigh Lifts*	42
27	Side Kicks - Inner Thigh Circles*	43
28	Side Kicks - Side Bicycle*	44
29	**SIDE KICKS - DOUBLE LEG LIFTS***	**45**
30	Side Kicks - Bicycle	33
31	Teaser 1	28
32	Teaser 2	41
33	Can Can	35
34	Mermaid	39
35	Seal With Beats	34
36	Pilates Push Up	36

*optional if needed by student

Side Kicks - Beats

Core 2:

- Baseline Variation: Goal Instructions

Advanced:

- Challenge Variation 1: Increase Repetitions

Super Advanced:

- Challenge Variation 2: Large Beats
  Use this variation before introducing Side Split on the Reformer.
- Challenge Variation 3: Alternating Accent
  To increase control.

Note: Beats is one of the optional Side Kicks, added only if the student needs it. The purpose noted is *for flabby legs. Also a gathering variation for a flexible person.*

The Order of Things
after Side Kicks - Beats

PERFORMANCE ORDER	EXERCISE	ADD NEXT #
1	Hundred	1
2	Roll Up	2
3	Single Leg Circle	3
4	Single Leg Circle Full	30
5	Roll Like a Ball	4
6	Single Leg Pull Bent	5
7	Double Leg Pull Bent	6
8	Single Leg Pull Straight	9
9	Double Leg Straight	24
10	Criss Cross	25
11	Spine Stretch Forward	7
12	Open Leg Rocker	18
13	Corkscrew Flat	26
14	Corkscrew Tail Off	32
15	Saw	15
16	Neck Roll	27
17	Swan Preparation	38
18	Single Leg Kick Back	14
19	Double Leg Kick Back	29
20	The Neck Pull	31
21	Spine Twist	40
22	Side Kicks - Front & Back	21
23	Side Kicks - Up & Down	20
24	Side Kicks - Small Circles	22
25	Side Kicks - Medium Circles*	37
26	Side Kicks - Inner Thigh Lifts*	42
27	Side Kicks - Inner Thigh Circles*	43
28	Side Kicks - Side Bicycle*	44
29	Side Kicks - Double Leg Lifts*	45
30	**SIDE KICKS - BEATS***	**46**
31	Side Kicks - Bicycle	33
32	Teaser 1	28
33	Teaser 2	41
34	Can Can	35
35	Mermaid	39
36	Seal With Beats	34
37	Pilates Push Up	36

*optional if needed by student

Side Kicks - Crosses

Add Next	47
Pages	187-188
Thread(s)	Stability 24 Side Bending 8

Core 2:
- Baseline Variation: Goal Instructions

Advanced:
- Challenge Variation 1: Increase Repetitions

Super Advanced:
- Challenge Variation 2: Large Beats
  Use this variation before introducing Side Splits on Reformer.
- Challenge Variation 3: Alternating Accent
  To increase control.

Note: Crosses is one of the optional Side Kicks that is added only if the student needs it. The purpose noted in Connection to Prior Exercise of the Thread: *"The crossing action increases work for the inner thighs and spinal Stabilization. This creates a greater challenge for balance."*

The Order of Things
after Side Kicks - Crosses

PERFORMANCE ORDER	EXERCISE	ADD NEXT #
1	Hundred	1
2	Roll Up	2
3	Single Leg Circle	3
4	Single Leg Circle Full	30
5	Roll Like a Ball	4
6	Single Leg Pull Bent	5
7	Double Leg Pull Bent	6
8	Single Leg Pull Straight	9
9	Double Leg Straight	24
10	Criss Cross	25
11	Spine Stretch Forward	7
12	Open Leg Rocker	18
13	Corkscrew Flat	26
14	Corkscrew Tail Off	32
15	Saw	15
16	Neck Roll	27
17	Swan Preparation	38
18	Single Leg Kick Back	14
19	Double Leg Kick Back	29
20	The Neck Pull	31
21	Spine Twist	40
22	Side Kicks - Front & Back	21
23	Side Kicks - Up & Down	20
24	Side Kicks - Small Circles	22
25	Side Kicks - Medium Circles*	37
26	Side Kicks - Inner Thigh Lifts*	42
27	Side Kicks - Inner Thigh Circles*	43
28	Side Kicks - Side Bicycle*	44
29	Side Kicks - Double Leg Lifts*	45
30	Side Kicks - Beats*	46
31	**SIDE KICKS - CROSSES***	**47**
32	Side Kicks - Bicycle	33
33	Teaser 1	28
34	Teaser 2	41
35	Can Can	35
36	Mermaid	39
37	Seal With Beats	34
38	Pilates Push Up	36

*optional if needed by student

Side Kicks - Large Circles

Add Next	48
Pages	173-174
Thread(s)	Stability 25
	Side Bending 9
	Extension 9

Core 2:

- Building Variation 1: Increase Repetitions
  To build strength
- Building Variation 2: Remove Pause in Circle When Heels Touch
  For the tense student to increase understanding of fluid movement.
- Baseline Variation: Goal Instructions
- Challenge Variation 3: Increase Dynamics
  To introduce dynamic action to the Side Kick Series.

Advanced:

- Challenge Variation 4: Lift Bottom Leg
  To prepare for the Single Leg Side Sit Up Series

The Order of Things
after Side Kicks - Large Circles

PERFORMANCE ORDER	EXERCISE	ADD NEXT #
1	Hundred	1
2	Roll Up	2
3	Single Leg Circle	3
4	Single Leg Circle Full	30
5	Roll Like a Ball	4
6	Single Leg Pull Bent	5
7	Double Leg Pull Bent	6
8	Single Leg Pull Straight	9
9	Double Leg Straight	24
10	Criss Cross	25
11	Spine Stretch Forward	7
12	Open Leg Rocker	18
13	Corkscrew Flat	26
14	Corkscrew Tail Off	32
15	Saw	15
16	Neck Roll	27
17	Swan Preparation	38
18	Single Leg Kick Back	14
19	Double Leg Kick Back	29
20	The Neck Pull	31
21	Spine Twist	40
22	Side Kicks - Front & Back	21
23	Side Kicks - Up & Down	20
24	Side Kicks - Small Circles	22
25	Side Kicks - Medium Circles*	37
26	**SIDE KICKS - LARGE CIRCLES**	**48**
27	Side Kicks - Inner Thigh Lifts*	42
28	Side Kicks - Inner Thigh Circles*	43
29	Side Kicks - Side Bicycle*	44
30	Side Kicks - Double Leg Lifts*	45
31	Side Kicks - Beats*	46
32	Side Kicks - Crosses*	47
33	Side Kicks - Bicycle	33
34	Teaser 1	28
35	Teaser 2	41
36	Can Can	35
37	Mermaid	39
38	Seal With Beats	34
39	Pilates Push Up	36

*optional if needed by student

Corkscrew Full

Core 2:
- Baseline Variation: Goal Instructions

The Order of Things
after Corkscrew Full

PERFORMANCE ORDER	EXERCISE	ADD NEXT #
1	Hundred	1
2	Roll Up	2
3	Single Leg Circle	3
4	Single Leg Circle Full	30
5	Roll Like a Ball	4
6	Single Leg Pull Bent	5
7	Double Leg Pull Bent	6
8	Single Leg Pull Straight	9
9	Double Leg Straight	24
10	Criss Cross	25
11	Spine Stretch Forward	7
12	Open Leg Rocker	18
13	Corkscrew Flat	26
14	Corkscrew Tail Off	32
15	**CORKSCREW FULL**	**49**
16	Saw	15
17	Neck Roll	27
18	Swan Preparation	38
19	Single Leg Kick Back	14
20	Double Leg Kick Back	29
21	The Neck Pull	31
22	Spine Twist	40
23	Side Kicks - Front & Back	21
24	Side Kicks - Up & Down	20
25	Side Kicks - Small Circles	22
26	Side Kicks - Medium Circles*	37
27	Side Kicks - Large Circles	48
28	Side Kicks - Inner Thigh Lifts*	42
29	Side Kicks - Inner Thigh Circles*	43
30	Side Kicks - Side Bicycle*	44
31	Side Kicks - Double Leg Lifts*	45
32	Side Kicks - Beats*	46
33	Side Kicks - Crosses*	47
34	Side Kicks - Bicycle	33
35	Teaser 1	28
36	Teaser 2	41
37	Can Can	35
38	Mermaid	39
39	Seal With Beats	34
40	Pilates Push Up	36

*optional if needed by student

Swimming

Add Next	50
Pages	233-235
Thread(s)	Stability 26 Extension 10

Core 2:

- Baseline Variation: Goal Instructions

Super Advanced:

- Challenge Variation 1: Vigorous Swim
- Challenge Variation 2: Head Lower and Lift
  To open the upper back and for the student who rocks upper back side to side.
- Challenge Variation 3: Turned Out Swim
  For the student who needs to work their bottom more or leg alignment requires turn out.

The Order of Things
after Swimming

PERFORMANCE ORDER	EXERCISE	ADD NEXT #
1	Hundred	1
2	Roll Up	2
3	Single Leg Circle	3
4	Single Leg Circle Full	30
5	Roll Like a Ball	4
6	Single Leg Pull Bent	5
7	Double Leg Pull Bent	6
8	Single Leg Pull Straight	9
9	Double Leg Straight	24
10	Criss Cross	25
11	Spine Stretch Forward	7
12	Open Leg Rocker	18
13	Corkscrew Flat	26
14	Corkscrew Tail Off	32
15	Corkscrew Full	49
16	Saw	15
17	Neck Roll	27
18	Swan Preparation	38
19	Single Leg Kick Back	14
20	Double Leg Kick Back	29
21	The Neck Pull	31
22	Spine Twist	40
23	Side Kicks - Front & Back	21
24	Side Kicks - Up & Down	20
25	Side Kicks - Small Circles	22
26	Side Kicks - Medium Circles*	37
27	Side Kicks - Large Circles	48
28	Side Kicks - Inner Thigh Lifts*	42
29	Side Kicks - Inner Thigh Circles*	43
30	Side Kicks - Side Bicycle*	44
31	Side Kicks - Double Leg Lifts*	45
32	Side Kicks - Beats*	46
33	Side Kicks - Crosses*	47
34	Side Kicks - Bicycle	33
35	Teaser 1	28
36	Teaser 2	41
37	Can Can	35
38	**SWIMMING**	**50**
39	Mermaid	39
40	Seal With Beats	34
41	Pilates Push Up	36

*optional if needed by student

Kneeling Side Kicks - Up & Down

Add Next	51
Pages	245 - 246
Thread(s)	Stability 27
	Side Bending 10

Core 2:
- Baseline Variation: Goal Instructions

Advanced:
- Challenge Variation 1: Increase Range of Motion
  To challenge stability.
- Challenge Variation 2: Add Accent
  To challenge stability.
- Challenge Variation 3: Vigorous Pace
  To challenge stability.

Super Advanced:
- Challenge Variation 4: Hold
  Teach before Star Side on the Reformer. To build strength and control.

The Order of Things
after Kneeling Side Kicks - Up & Down

PERFORMANCE ORDER	EXERCISE	ADD NEXT #
1	Hundred	1
2	Roll Up	2
3	Single Leg Circle	3
4	Single Leg Circle Full	30
5	Roll Like a Ball	4
6	Single Leg Pull Bent	5
7	Double Leg Pull Bent	6
8	Single Leg Pull Straight	9
9	Double Leg Straight	24
10	Criss Cross	25
11	Spine Stretch Forward	7
12	Open Leg Rocker	18
13	Corkscrew Flat	26
14	Corkscrew Tail Off	32
15	Corkscrew Full	49
16	Saw	15
17	Neck Roll	27
18	Swan Preparation	38
19	Single Leg Kick Back	14
20	Double Leg Kick Back	29
21	The Neck Pull	31
22	Spine Twist	40
23	Side Kicks - Front & Back	21
24	Side Kicks - Up & Down	20
25	Side Kicks - Small Circles	22
26	Side Kicks - Medium Circles*	37
27	Side Kicks - Large Circles	48
28	Side Kicks - Inner Thigh Lifts*	42
29	Side Kicks - Inner Thigh Circles*	43
30	Side Kicks - Side Bicycle*	44
31	Side Kicks - Double Leg Lifts*	45
32	Side Kicks - Beats*	46
33	Side Kicks - Crosses*	47
34	Side Kicks - Bicycle	33
35	Teaser 1	28
36	Teaser 2	41
37	Can Can	35
38	Swimming	50
39	**KNEELING SIDE KICKS - UP & DOWN**	**51**
40	Mermaid	39
41	Seal With Beats	34
42	Pilates Push Up	36

*optional if needed by student

Kneeling Side Kicks - Front & Back

Core 2:
- Baseline Variation: Goal Instructions

Advanced:
- Challenge Variation 1: Increase Range of Motion
  To challenge stability.
- Challenge Variation 2: Add Accent
  To challenge stability.
- Challenge Variation 3: Vigorous Pace
  To challenge stability.

Super Advanced:
- Challenge Variation 4: Hold
  Teach before Star Front & Back on Reformer. Builds strength and control.
- Challenge Variation 5: Old Fashioned
  Teach before Star Old Fashioned on the Reformer. Builds strength and control.

The Order of Things
after Kneeling Side Kicks - Front & Back

PERFORMANCE ORDER	EXERCISE	ADD NEXT #
1	Hundred	1
2	Roll Up	2
3	Single Leg Circle	3
4	Single Leg Circle Full	30
5	Roll Like a Ball	4
6	Single Leg Pull Bent	5
7	Double Leg Pull Bent	6
8	Single Leg Pull Straight	9
9	Double Leg Straight	24
10	Criss Cross	25
11	Spine Stretch Forward	7
12	Open Leg Rocker	18
13	Corkscrew Flat	26
14	Corkscrew Tail Off	32
15	Corkscrew Full	49
16	Saw	15
17	Neck Roll	27
18	Swan Preparation	38
19	Single Leg Kick Back	14
20	Double Leg Kick Back	29
21	The Neck Pull	31
22	Spine Twist	40
23	Side Kicks - Front & Back	21
24	Side Kicks - Up & Down	20
25	Side Kicks - Small Circles	22
26	Side Kicks - Medium Circles*	37
27	Side Kicks - Large Circles	48
28	Side Kicks - Inner Thigh Lifts*	42
29	Side Kicks - Inner Thigh Circles*	43
30	Side Kicks - Side Bicycle*	44
31	Side Kicks - Double Leg Lifts*	45
32	Side Kicks - Beats*	46
33	Side Kicks - Crosses*	47
34	Side Kicks - Bicycle	33
35	Teaser 1	28
36	Teaser 2	41
37	Can Can	35
38	Swimming	50
39	**KNEELING SIDE KICKS - FRONT & BACK**	**52**
40	Kneeling Side Kicks - Up & Down	51
41	Mermaid	39
42	Seal With Beats	34
43	Pilates Push Up	36

*optional if needed by student

Side Kicks - Grand Circles

Add Next	53
Pages	193-195
Thread(s)	Stability 29
	Side Bending 11
	Extension 12

Core 2:
- Baseline Variation: Goal Instructions

Advanced:
- Challenge Variation 1: Increase Repetitions
- Unofficial Challenge Variation (from Teaching Note): Hands Behind Head

Super Advanced:
- Note: Use Side Split transition (see Transition Option "Split Change Transition", page 162)

Note: Grand Circles is one of the optional Side Kicks, added only if the student needs it. A purpose noted in Side Kick Series Set Up & Focus is *a freeing variation for a student who is a tight and tense person.*

This completes the Core Level sequence.

The Order of Things
after Side Kicks - Grand Circles

PERFORMANCE ORDER	EXERCISE	ADD NEXT #
1	Hundred	1
2	Roll Up	2
3	Single Leg Circle	3
4	Single Leg Circle Full	30
5	Roll Like a Ball	4
6	Single Leg Pull Bent	5
7	Double Leg Pull Bent	6
8	Single Leg Pull Straight	9
9	Double Leg Straight	24
10	Criss Cross	25
11	Spine Stretch Forward	7
12	Open Leg Rocker	18
13	Corkscrew Flat	26
14	Corkscrew Tail Off	32
15	Corkscrew Full	49
16	Saw	15
17	Neck Roll	27
18	Swan Preparation	38
19	Single Leg Kick Back	14
20	Double Leg Kick Back	29
21	The Neck Pull	31
22	Spine Twist	40
23	Side Kicks - Front & Back	21
24	Side Kicks - Up & Down	20
25	Side Kicks - Small Circles	22
26	Side Kicks - Medium Circles*	37
27	Side Kicks - Large Circles	48
28	Side Kicks - Inner Thigh Lifts*	42
29	Side Kicks - Inner Thigh Circles*	43
30	Side Kicks - Side Bicycle*	44
31	Side Kicks - Double Leg Lifts*	45
32	Side Kicks - Beats*	46
33	Side Kicks - Crosses*	47
34	Side Kicks - Bicycle	33
35	**SIDE KICKS - GRAND CIRCLES ***	**53**
36	Teaser 1	28
37	Teaser 2	41
38	Can Can	35
39	Swimming	50
40	Kneeling Side Kicks - Front & Back	52
41	Kneeling Side Kicks - Up & Down	51
42	Mermaid	39
43	Seal With Beats	34
44	Pilates Push Up	36

*optional if needed by student

Roll Over

Add Next	54
Pages	41-44
Thread(s)	Articulation 10

Advanced:

- Building Variation 1: Float Feet
  To build stretch and control.
- Baseline Version: Goal Instructions
- Challenge Variation 2: Pointed Feet
  To increase stretch for the front of legs and lengthen out of hips.
- Challenge Variation 3: Flex Point Flex
  To increase stretch for back of legs and lower back.

Super Advanced:

- Challenge Variation 4: Full Overhead
  For deep stretch, strength, control and spinal opening.
- Challenge Variation 5: Reverse Breathing
  To work lungs and control.
- Challenge Variation 6: Wide Circles
  To relax hips.

The Order of Things
after Roll Over

PERFORMANCE ORDER	EXERCISE	ADD NEXT #
1	Hundred	1
2	Roll Up	2
3	**ROLL OVER**	**54**
4	Single Leg Circle	3
5	Single Leg Circle Full	30
6	Roll Like a Ball	4
7	Single Leg Pull Bent	5
8	Double Leg Pull Bent	6
9	Single Leg Pull Straight	9
10	Double Leg Straight	24
11	Criss Cross	25
12	Spine Stretch Forward	7
13	Open Leg Rocker	18
14	Corkscrew Flat	26
15	Corkscrew Tail Off	32
16	Corkscrew Full	49
17	Saw	15
18	Neck Roll	27
19	Swan Preparation	38
20	Single Leg Kick Back	14
21	Double Leg Kick Back	29
22	The Neck Pull	31
23	Spine Twist	40
24	Side Kicks - Front & Back	21
25	Side Kicks - Up & Down	20
26	Side Kicks - Small Circles	22
27	Side Kicks - Medium Circles*	37
28	Side Kicks - Large Circles	48
29	Side Kicks - Inner Thigh Lifts*	42
30	Side Kicks - Inner Thigh Circles*	43
31	Side Kicks - Side Bicycle*	44
32	Side Kicks - Double Leg Lifts*	45
33	Side Kicks - Beats*	46
34	Side Kicks - Crosses*	47
35	Side Kicks - Bicycle	33
36	Side Kicks - Grand Circles *	53
37	Teaser 1	28
38	Teaser 2	41
39	Can Can	35
40	Swimming	50
41	Kneeling Side Kicks - Front & Back	52
42	Kneeling Side Kicks - Up & Down	51
43	Mermaid	39
44	Seal With Beats	34
45	Pilates Push Up	36

*optional if needed by student

Teaser 3

Add Next	55
Pages	221-226
Thread(s)	Articulation 11

Advanced:

- Building Variation 1: Arms by Side
  Palms up to keep shoulders engaged, palms down to connect to the back body.
- Baseline Variation: Goal Instructions
- Challenge Variation 2: Arms to Ceiling Roll Back
  Teach before Up Stretch on the Reformer.
- Challenge Variation 3: Arms to Ceiling Reach Back
  Teach before Up Stretch on the Reformer.
- Challenge Variation 4: Arm by Ears
  Teach before Up Stretch on the Reformer.

Super Advanced:

- Challenge Variation 5: Toe Touches
  Teach before Hip Circles (Add Next #56)
- Challenge Variation 6: Open Circle Legs & Arms in Opposition
  To build coordination.
- Challenge Variation 7: Twisting
  Teach after Hip Circles (Add Next #56) and before Snake & Twist on the Reformer.
- Challenge Variation 8: Walking
  To build coordination and abdominal strength.
- Challenge Variation 9: Beat Legs
  To increase connection to the Trinity.
- Challenge Variation 10: Close Envelope – Open Envelope
  Teach before Hip Circles (Add Next #56)
- Challenge Variation 11: Twisting 2
  Teach after Hip Circles (Add Next #56) and before Snake & Twist on the Reformer.
- Challenge Variation 12: Pelvic Stability
  To build the stability of the pelvis.
- Challenge Variation 13: Rowing Series
  To build abdominal, back and arm connection to the chest.
- Challenge Variation 14: Shaving
- Challenge Variation 15: Swan Dive Teaser Combination

The Order of Things
after Teaser 3

PERFORMANCE ORDER	EXERCISE	ADD NEXT #
1	Hundred	1
2	Roll Up	2
3	Roll Over	54
4	Single Leg Circle	3
5	Single Leg Circle Full	30
6	Roll Like a Ball	4
7	Single Leg Pull Bent	5
8	Double Leg Pull Bent	6
9	Single Leg Pull Straight	9
10	Double Leg Straight	24
11	Criss Cross	25
12	Spine Stretch Forward	7
13	Open Leg Rocker	18
14	Corkscrew Flat	26
15	Corkscrew Tail Off	32
16	Corkscrew Full	49
17	Saw	15
18	Neck Roll	27
19	Swan Preparation	38
20	Single Leg Kick Back	14
21	Double Leg Kick Back	29
22	The Neck Pull	31
23	Spine Twist	40
24	Side Kicks - Front & Back	21
25	Side Kicks - Up & Down	20
26	Side Kicks - Small Circles	22
27	Side Kicks - Medium Circles*	37
28	Side Kicks - Large Circles	48
29	Side Kicks - Inner Thigh Lifts*	42
30	Side Kicks - Inner Thigh Circles*	43
31	Side Kicks - Side Bicycle*	44
32	Side Kicks - Double Leg Lifts*	45
33	Side Kicks - Beats*	46
34	Side Kicks - Crosses*	47
35	Side Kicks - Bicycle	33
36	Side Kicks - Grand Circles *	53
37	Teaser 1	28
38	Teaser 2	41
39	**TEASER 3**	**55**
40	Can Can	35
41	Swimming	50
42	Kneeling Side Kicks - Front & Back	52
43	Kneeling Side Kicks - Up & Down	51
44	Mermaid	39
45	Seal With Beats	34
46	Pilates Push Up	36

*optional if needed by student

Hip Circles

Add Next	56
Pages	229-232
Thread(s)	Twisting 11

Advanced:

- Building Variation 1: Bent Arms Mat
  To introduce the Hip Circles or for the student who arches the lower back when arms are fully extended.
- Building Variation 2: Bent Elbows
  For the student who hyperextends and locks their elbows or has wrist issues.
- Building Variation 3: Lifted Single Leg Tick Tock 1
  For the student who side bends or swivels the hips instead of twisting.
- Building Variation 4: Lifted Single Leg Tick Tock 2
  For the student who side bends or swivels the hips instead of twisting.
- Building Variation 5: Windshield Wiper
  For the student who side bends or swivels the hips instead of twisting.
- Baseline Variation: Goal Instructions

Super Advanced:

- Challenge Variation 6: Teacher's Stretch
  To add stretch to the strength.
- Challenge Variation 7: Leg Toss Side to Side
  To add strength and control.
- Challenge Variation 8: Touch & Pause
  To add strength to the stretch.
- Challenge Variation 9: Sweep
  To create fluid movement.

Note: once Hip Circles have been taught consider if student is ready for Challenge Variation 2 of Teaser Two (*Add Next #41*) - Circles in Opposition.

Note: The Can Can (Add Next #35) is the introductory exercise to Hip Circles. So once Hip Circles gets added, it replaces the Can Can in the Performance Order.

The Order of Things
after Hip Circles

PERFORMANCE ORDER	EXERCISE	ADD NEXT #
1	Hundred	1
2	Roll Up	2
3	Roll Over	54
4	Single Leg Circle	3
5	Single Leg Circle Full	30
6	Roll Like a Ball	4
7	Single Leg Pull Bent	5
8	Double Leg Pull Bent	6
9	Single Leg Pull Straight	9
10	Double Leg Straight	24
11	Criss Cross	25
12	Spine Stretch Forward	7
13	Open Leg Rocker	18
14	Corkscrew Flat	26
15	Corkscrew Tail Off	32
16	Corkscrew Full	49
17	Saw	15
18	Neck Roll	27
19	Swan Preparation	38
20	Single Leg Kick Back	14
21	Double Leg Kick Back	29
22	Neck Pull	31
23	Spine Twist	40
24	Side Kicks - Front & Back	21
25	Side Kicks - Up & Down	20
26	Side Kicks - Small Circles	22
27	Side Kicks - Medium Circles*	37
28	Side Kicks - Large Circles	48
29	Side Kicks - Inner Thigh Lifts*	42
30	Side Kicks - Inner Thigh Circles*	43
31	Side Kicks - Side Bicycle*	44
32	Side Kicks - Double Leg Lifts*	45
33	Side Kicks - Beats*	46
34	Side Kicks - Crosses*	47
35	Side Kicks - Bicycle	33
36	Side Kicks - Grand Circles *	53
37	Teaser 1	28
38	Teaser 2	41
39	Teaser 3	55
40	**HIP CIRCLES**	**56**
41	Swimming	50
42	Kneeling Side Kicks - Front & Back	52
43	Kneeling Side Kicks - Up & Down	51
44	Mermaid	39
45	Seal With Beats	34
46	Pilates Push Up	36

*optional if needed by student

Leg Pull Front

Add Next	57
Pages	237-238
Thread(s)	Stability 30 Extension 13

Advanced:
- Unofficial Building Variation (from Teaching): No Pulse
- Baseline Variation: Goal Instructions

Super Advanced:
- Challenge Variation 1: Leg High
  Teach before Elephant on Top on the Reformer.
- Challenge Variation 2: Leg Side
  Teach before Tendon Stretch to the Side on the Reformer.
- Challenge Variation 3: Leg Back & Side Combo
  Teach before Tendon Stretch Combination on the Reformer.
- Challenge Variation 4: Lifted Arm
  To challenge balance.

Note: Teach Leg Pull Front before Challenge Variations 3 and 4 of Pilates Push Up (*Add Next #36)*

The Order of Things
after Leg Pull Front

PERFORMANCE ORDER	EXERCISE	ADD NEXT #
1	Hundred	1
2	Roll Up	2
3	Roll Over	54
4	Single Leg Circle	3
5	Single Leg Circle Full	30
6	Roll Like a Ball	4
7	Single Leg Pull Bent	5
8	Double Leg Pull Bent	6
9	Single Leg Pull Straight	9
10	Double Leg Straight	24
11	Criss Cross	25
12	Spine Stretch Forward	7
13	Open Leg Rocker	18
14	Corkscrew Flat	26
15	Corkscrew Tail Off	32
16	Corkscrew Full	49
17	Saw	15
18	Neck Roll	27
19	Swan Preparation	38
20	Single Leg Kick Back	14
21	Double Leg Kick Back	29
22	The Neck Pull	31
23	Spine Twist	40
24	Side Kicks - Front & Back	21
25	Side Kicks - Up & Down	20
26	Side Kicks - Small Circles	22
27	Side Kicks - Medium Circles*	37
28	Side Kicks - Large Circles	48
29	Side Kicks - Inner Thigh Lifts*	42
30	Side Kicks - Inner Thigh Circles*	43
31	Side Kicks - Side Bicycle*	44
32	Side Kicks - Double Leg Lifts*	45
33	Side Kicks - Beats*	46
34	Side Kicks - Crosses*	47
35	Side Kicks - Bicycle	33
36	Side Kicks - Grand Circles *	53
37	Teaser 1	28
38	Teaser 2	41
39	Teaser 3	55
40	Hip Circles	56
41	Swimming	50
42	**LEG PULL FRONT**	**57**
43	Kneeling Side Kicks - Front & Back	52
44	Kneeling Side Kicks - Up & Down	51
45	Mermaid	39
46	Seal With Beats	34
47	Pilates Push Up	36

*optional if needed by student

Leg Pull Back

Add Next	58
Pages	239-240
Thread(s)	Stability 31 Extension 14

Advanced:

- Baseline Variation: Goal Instructions
- Unofficial Challenge Variation (in Teaching): Point Up, Flex Down
  For a greater stretch.
- Unofficial Challenge Variation (in Goal Instructions): Flexed Feet
  To help back body connection.

Super Advanced:

- Challenge Variation 1: Leg Side
  To prepare for Fan Kicks on the Control Balance Series on the Reformer.
- Challenge Variation 2: Leg Side & Up
  In preparation for Control Balance Series on the Reformer.

The Order of Things
after Leg Pull Back

PERFORMANCE ORDER	EXERCISE	ADD NEXT #
1	Hundred	1
2	Roll Up	2
3	Roll Over	54
4	Single Leg Circle	3
5	Single Leg Circle Full	30
6	Roll Like a Ball	4
7	Single Leg Pull Bent	5
8	Double Leg Pull Bent	6
9	Single Leg Pull Straight	9
10	Double Leg Straight	24
11	Criss Cross	25
12	Spine Stretch Forward	7
13	Open Leg Rocker	18
14	Corkscrew Flat	26
15	Corkscrew Tail Off	32
16	Corkscrew Full	49
17	Saw	15
18	Neck Roll	27
19	Swan Preparation	38
20	Single Leg Kick Back	14
21	Double Leg Kick Back	29
22	Neck Pull	31
23	Spine Twist	40
24	Side Kicks - Front & Back	21
25	Side Kicks - Up & Down	20
26	Side Kicks - Small Circles	22
27	Side Kicks - Medium Circles*	37
28	Side Kicks - Large Circles	48
29	Side Kicks - Inner Thigh Lifts*	42
30	Side Kicks - Inner Thigh Circles*	43
31	Side Kicks - Side Bicycle*	44
32	Side Kicks - Double Leg Lifts*	45
33	Side Kicks - Beats*	46
34	Side Kicks - Crosses*	47
35	Side Kicks - Bicycle	33
36	Side Kicks - Grand Circles *	53
37	Teaser 1	28
38	Teaser 2	41
39	Teaser 3	55
40	Hip Circles	56
41	Swimming	50
42	Leg Pull Front	57
43	**LEG PULL BACK**	**58**
44	Kneeling Side Kicks - Front & Back	52
45	Kneeling Side Kicks - Up & Down	51
46	Mermaid	39
47	Seal With Beats	34
48	Pilates Push Up	36

*optional if needed by student

Thigh Stretch

Add Next	59
Pages	129-132
Thread(s)	Stability 32

Advanced:
- Building Variation 1: Hold Heels
  To open the front of the hips or for a student who sits towards the heels when they hinge back.
- Baseline Variation: Goal Instructions
- Challenge Variation 2: Long Spine – Head Up (Neck Straight)
  To develop Flack Back on Short Box on the Reformer. Also noted as the goal in the Goal Instructions.
- Challenge Variation 3: Reverse Thigh Stretch
  Open front of the hips and challenge strength.

Super Advanced:
- Challenge Variation 4: Legs Together
  To develop Legs Together Chest Expansion on the Reformer and Rocking (Add Next #67)
- Challenge Variation 5: Weighted Bar
  To prepare for Breathing with Straps on the Reformer, Rocking (Add Next #67) and High Bridge (Add Next #77)
- Challenge Variation 6: Full Release
  To develop Back Bend Bar Up & Down on the Reformer, and High Bridge on the Mat (Add Next #77)
- Unofficial Challenge Variation 6+: Full Release with Weighted Bar

The Order of Things
after Thigh Stretch

PERFORMANCE ORDER	EXERCISE	ADD NEXT #
1	Hundred	1
2	Roll Up	2
3	Roll Over	54
4	Single Leg Circle	3
5	Single Leg Circle Full	30
6	Roll Like a Ball	4
7	Single Leg Pull Bent	5
8	Double Leg Pull Bent	6
9	Single Leg Pull Straight	9
10	Double Leg Straight	24
11	Criss Cross	25
12	Spine Stretch Forward	7
13	Open Leg Rocker	18
14	Corkscrew Flat	26
15	Corkscrew Tail Off	32
16	Corkscrew Full	49
17	Saw	15
18	Neck Roll	27
19	Swan Preparation	38
20	Single Leg Kick Back	14
21	Double Leg Kick Back	29
22	**THIGH STRETCH**	**59**
23	The Neck Pull	31
24	Spine Twist	40
25	Side Kicks - Front & Back	21
26	Side Kicks - Up & Down	20
27	Side Kicks - Small Circles	22
28	Side Kicks - Medium Circles*	37
29	Side Kicks - Large Circles	48
30	Side Kicks - Inner Thigh Lifts*	42
31	Side Kicks - Inner Thigh Circles*	43
32	Side Kicks - Side Bicycle*	44
33	Side Kicks - Double Leg Lifts*	45
34	Side Kicks - Beats*	46
35	Side Kicks - Crosses*	47
36	Side Kicks - Bicycle	33
37	Side Kicks - Grand Circles *	53
38	Teaser 1	28
39	Teaser 2	41
40	Teaser 3	55
41	Hip Circles	56
42	Swimming	50
43	Leg Pull Front	57
44	Leg Pull Back	58
45	Kneeling Side Kicks - Front & Back	52
46	Kneeling Side Kicks - Up & Down	51
47	Mermaid	39
48	Seal With Beats	34
49	Pilates Push Up	36

*optional if needed by student

Side Bend

Add Next	60
Pages	261-264
Thread(s)	Side Bending 12

Advanced:

- Unofficial Building Variations in Teaching instructions:
  - Top foot in front of bottom foot
  - Without lowering bottom side
- Baseline Variation: Goal Instructions

Super Advanced:

- Challenge Variation 2: Deep Bend
  Teach before Snake & Twist (Add Next #61)
- Challenge Variation 3: Hip Lower
  Teach before Snake on Reformer.
- Challenge Variation 4: Arm Bend
  Teach before Snake Arm Bend on Reformer.
- Challenge Variation 5: Side Star
  Teach before Star on the Reformer.
- Challenge Variation 6: Star Front & Back
  Teach before Star Front & Back on the Reformer.
- Challenge Variation 7: Star Old Fashioned
  Teach before Star old Fashioned on the Reformer.

Performance Order Note 1: Challenge Variations can replace the Side Bend or a single repetition can be added as the third Side Bend.

Performance Order Note 2: when Side Bend is added, Mermaid is omitted from the Performance Order.

The Order of Things
after Side Bend

PERFORMANCE ORDER	EXERCISE	ADD NEXT #
1	Hundred	1
2	Roll Up	2
3	Roll Over	54
4	Single Leg Circle	3
5	Single Leg Circle Full	30
6	Roll Like a Ball	4
7	Single Leg Pull Bent	5
8	Double Leg Pull Bent	6
9	Single Leg Pull Straight	9
10	Double Leg Straight	24
11	Criss Cross	25
12	Spine Stretch Forward	7
13	Open Leg Rocker	18
14	Corkscrew Flat	26
15	Corkscrew Tail Off	32
16	Corkscrew Full	49
17	Saw	15
18	Neck Roll	27
19	Swan Preparation	38
20	Single Leg Kick Back	14
21	Double Leg Kick Back	29
22	Thigh Stretch	59
23	The Neck Pull	31
24	Spine Twist	40
25	Side Kicks - Front & Back	21
26	Side Kicks - Up & Down	20
27	Side Kicks - Small Circles	22
28	Side Kicks - Medium Circles*	37
29	Side Kicks - Large Circles	48
30	Side Kicks - Inner Thigh Lifts*	42
31	Side Kicks - Inner Thigh Circles*	43
32	Side Kicks - Side Bicycle*	44
33	Side Kicks - Double Leg Lifts*	45
34	Side Kicks - Beats*	46
35	Side Kicks - Crosses*	47
36	Side Kicks - Bicycle	33
37	Side Kicks - Grand Circles *	53
38	Teaser 1	28
39	Teaser 2	41
40	Teaser 3	55
41	Hip Circles	56
42	Swimming	50
43	Leg Pull Front	57
44	Leg Pull Back	58
45	Kneeling Side Kicks - Front & Back	52
46	Kneeling Side Kicks - Up & Down	51
47	**SIDE BEND**	**60**
48	Seal With Beats	34
49	Pilates Push Up	36

*optional if needed by student

Snake & Twist

Add Next	61
Pages	257-260
Thread(s)	Side Bending 13
	Extension 15
	Twisting 12
	Articulation 12

Advanced:

- Baseline Variation (Snake): Goal Instructions - Snake
- Unofficial Challenge Variation (in Teaching): Stack legs.
- Challenge Variation 1: One Hand
  To develop side body stabilization and balance.
- Unofficial Building Variation (in Teaching Snake & Twist): Top foot in front
- Unofficial Building Variation (in Teaching Snake & Twist): Without lowering bottom side.
- Baseline Variation (Snake & Twist): Goal Instructions - Snake & Twist

Super Advanced:

- Replace Side Bend with Snake & Twist and add Side Bend to the last repetition of Shake & Twist

The Order of Things
after Snake & Twist

PERFORMANCE ORDER	EXERCISE	ADD NEXT #
1	Hundred	1
2	Roll Up	2
3	Roll Over	54
4	Single Leg Circle	3
5	Single Leg Circle Full	30
6	Roll Like a Ball	4
7	Single Leg Pull Bent	5
8	Double Leg Pull Bent	6
9	Single Leg Pull Straight	9
10	Double Leg Straight	24
11	Criss Cross	25
12	Spine Stretch Forward	7
13	Open Leg Rocker	18
14	Corkscrew Flat	26
15	Corkscrew Tail Off	32
16	Corkscrew Full	49
17	Saw	15
18	Neck Roll	27
19	Swan Preparation	38
20	Single Leg Kick Back	14
21	Double Leg Kick Back	29
22	Thigh Stretch	59
23	The Neck Pull	31
24	Spine Twist	40
25	Side Kicks - Front & Back	21
26	Side Kicks - Up & Down	20
27	Side Kicks - Small Circles	22
28	Side Kicks - Medium Circles*	37
29	Side Kicks - Large Circles	48
30	Side Kicks - Inner Thigh Lifts*	42
31	Side Kicks - Inner Thigh Circles*	43
32	Side Kicks - Side Bicycle*	44
33	Side Kicks - Double Leg Lifts*	45
34	Side Kicks - Beats*	46
35	Side Kicks - Crosses*	47
36	Side Kicks - Bicycle	33
37	Side Kicks - Grand Circles *	53
38	Teaser 1	28
39	Teaser 2	41
40	Teaser 3	55
41	Hip Circles	56
42	Swimming	50
43	Leg Pull Front	57
44	Leg Pull Back	58
45	Kneeling Side Kicks - Front & Back	52
46	Kneeling Side Kicks - Up & Down	51
47	**SNAKE & TWIST**	**61**
48	Side Bend	60
49	Seal With Beats	34
50	Pilates Push Up	36

*optional if needed by student

Jackknife

Add Next	62
Pages	155-157
Thread(s)	Articulation 13

Advanced:
- Building Variation 1: Tailbone Off
  To introduce the Jackknife.
- Building Variation 2: Legs Overhead to 45-Degrees
  Introduce this way to prevent collapsing of the waistline.
- Baseline Variation: Goal Instructions

Super Advanced:
- Challenge Variation 3: Legs to Floor
  In preparation for the Boomerang
- Challenge Variation 4: Extra Touch
  To build spinal strength, stability and the Trinity needed in leg lifting exercises.
- Challenge Variation 5: Hand Lift
  In preparation for Rolling to Standing on the Control Balances (Add Next #69

The Order of Things
after Jackknife

PERFORMANCE ORDER	EXERCISE	ADD NEXT #
1	Hundred	1
2	Roll Up	2
3	Roll Over	54
4	Single Leg Circle	3
5	Single Leg Circle Full	30
6	Roll Like a Ball	4
7	Single Leg Pull Bent	5
8	Double Leg Pull Bent	6
9	Single Leg Pull Straight	9
10	Double Leg Straight	24
11	Criss Cross	25
12	Spine Stretch Forward	7
13	Open Leg Rocker	18
14	Corkscrew Flat	26
15	Corkscrew Tail Off	32
16	Corkscrew Full	49
17	Saw	15
18	Neck Roll	27
19	Swan Preparation	38
20	Single Leg Kick Back	14
21	Double Leg Kick Back	29
22	Thigh Stretch	59
23	The Neck Pull	31

The Order of Things
after Jackknife

PERFORMANCE ORDER	EXERCISE	ADD NEXT #
24	Spine Twist	40
25	**JACKKNIFE**	**62**
26	Side Kicks - Front & Back	21
27	Side Kicks - Up & Down	20
28	Side Kicks - Small Circles	22
29	Side Kicks - Medium Circles*	37
30	Side Kicks - Large Circles	48
31	Side Kicks - Inner Thigh Lifts*	42
32	Side Kicks - Inner Thigh Circles*	43
33	Side Kicks - Side Bicycle*	44
34	Side Kicks - Double Leg Lifts*	45
35	Side Kicks - Beats*	46
36	Side Kicks - Crosses*	47
37	Side Kicks - Bicycle	33
38	Side Kicks - Grand Circles *	53
39	Teaser 1	28
40	Teaser 2	41
41	Teaser 3	55
42	Hip Circles	56
43	Swimming	50
44	Leg Pull Front	57
45	Leg Pull Back	58
46	Kneeling Side Kicks - Front & Back	52
47	Kneeling Side Kicks - Up & Down	51
48	Snake & Twist	61
49	Side Bend	60
50	Seal With Beats	34
51	Pilates Push Up	36

*optional if needed by student

Corkscrew Twist

Add Next	63
Pages	105-106
Thread(s)	Twisting 13

Advanced:

- Baseline Variation: Goal Instructions

Super Advanced:

- Challenge Variation 1: Corkscrew 90-Degree Old Fashioned
  Challenges the lift of the waist and Powerhouse control.

The Order of Things
after Corkscrew Twist

PERFORMANCE ORDER	EXERCISE	ADD NEXT #
1	Hundred	1
2	Roll Up	2
3	Roll Over	54
4	Single Leg Circle	3
5	Single Leg Circle Full	30
6	Roll Like a Ball	4
7	Single Leg Pull Bent	5
8	Double Leg Pull Bent	6
9	Single Leg Pull Straight	9
10	Double Leg Straight	24
11	Criss Cross	25
12	Spine Stretch Forward	7
13	Open Leg Rocker	18
14	Corkscrew Flat	26
15	Corkscrew Tail Off	32
16	Corkscrew Full	49
17	**CORKSCREW TWIST**	**63**
18	Saw	15
19	Neck Roll	27
20	Swan Preparation	38
21	Single Leg Kick Back	14
22	Double Leg Kick Back	29
23	Thigh Stretch	59
24	The Neck Pull	31
25	Spine Twist	40
26	Jackknife	62

The Order of Things
after Corkscrew Twist

PERFORMANCE ORDER	EXERCISE	ADD NEXT #
27	Side Kicks - Front & Back	21
28	Side Kicks - Up & Down	20
29	Side Kicks - Small Circles	22
30	Side Kicks - Medium Circles*	37
31	Side Kicks - Large Circles	48
32	Side Kicks - Inner Thigh Lifts*	42
33	Side Kicks - Inner Thigh Circles*	43
34	Side Kicks - Side Bicycle*	44
35	Side Kicks - Double Leg Lifts*	45
36	Side Kicks - Beats*	46
37	Side Kicks - Crosses*	47
38	Side Kicks - Bicycle	33
39	Side Kicks - Grand Circles *	53
40	Teaser 1	28
41	Teaser 2	41
42	Teaser 3	55
43	Hip Circles	56
44	Swimming	50
45	Leg Pull Front	57
46	Leg Pull Back	58
47	Kneeling Side Kicks - Front & Back	52
48	Kneeling Side Kicks - Up & Down	51
49	Snake & Twist	61
50	Side Bend	60
51	Seal With Beats	34
52	Pilates Push Up	36

*optional, if needed by student

Tick Tock

Add Next	64
Pages	107-108
Thread(s)	Twisting 14

Advanced:
- Baseline Variation: Goal Instructions

Super Advanced:
- Challenge Variation 1: Vigorous Tempo
  To introduce dynamic action into the workout.
- Challenge Variation 2: Teacher Throws Legs Side-to-Side
  To increase abdominal control and strength.
- Challenge Variation 3: Teacher Throws Legs Three Directions
  To increase abdominal control and strength. To prepare the Student for the unexpected and train the first muscular response of "catching themselves" with their stomach.

Performance Order Note (in Teaching section): "Sometimes a small ROM Tick Tock can be taught after Corkscrew Flat and before Corkscrew Tail Off."

The Order of Things
after Tick Tock

PERFORMANCE ORDER	EXERCISE	ADD NEXT #
1	Hundred	1
2	Roll Up	2
3	Roll Over	54
4	Single Leg Circle	3
5	Single Leg Circle Full	30
6	Roll Like a Ball	4
7	Single Leg Pull Bent	5
8	Double Leg Pull Bent	6
9	Single Leg Pull Straight	9
10	Double Leg Straight	24
11	Criss Cross	25
12	Spine Stretch Forward	7
13	Open Leg Rocker	18
14	Corkscrew Flat	26
15	Corkscrew Tail Off	32
16	Corkscrew Full	49
17	Corkscrew Twist	63
18	**TICK TOCK**	**64**
19	Saw	15

The Order of Things
after Tick Tock

PERFORMANCE ORDER	EXERCISE	ADD NEXT #
20	Neck Roll	27
21	Swan Preparation	38
22	Single Leg Kick Back	14
23	Double Leg Kick Back	29
24	Thigh Stretch	59
25	The Neck Pull	31
26	Spine Twist	40
27	Jackknife	62
28	Side Kicks - Front & Back	21
29	Side Kicks - Up & Down	20
30	Side Kicks - Small Circles	22
31	Side Kicks - Medium Circles*	37
32	Side Kicks - Large Circles	48
33	Side Kicks - Inner Thigh Lifts*	42
34	Side Kicks - Inner Thigh Circles*	43
35	Side Kicks - Side Bicycle*	44
36	Side Kicks - Double Leg Lifts*	45
37	Side Kicks - Beats*	46
38	Side Kicks - Crosses*	47
39	Side Kicks - Bicycle	33
40	Side Kicks - Grand Circles *	53
41	Teaser 1	28
42	Teaser 2	41
43	Teaser 3	55
44	Hip Circles	56
45	Swimming	50
46	Leg Pull Front	57
47	Leg Pull Back	58
48	Kneeling Side Kicks - Front & Back	52
49	Kneeling Side Kicks - Up & Down	51
50	Snake & Twist	61
51	Side Bend	60
52	Seal With Beats	34
53	Pilates Push Up	36

*optional, if needed by student

Kneeling Side Kicks - Circles

Add Next	65
Pages	247-248
Thread(s)	Stability 33
	Extension 16
	Side Bending 14

Advanced:

- Baseline Variation: Goal Instructions
- Challenge Variation 1: Increase Range of Motion
  To challenge stability.
- Challenge Variation 2: Add Accent
- Challenge Variation 3: Vigorous Pace
  To challenge Stability.

Super Advanced:

- Challenge Variation 4: Hold
  Teach before Star Old Fashioned on the Reformer.

The Order of Things
after Kneeling Side Kicks - Circles

PERFORMANCE ORDER	EXERCISE	ADD NEXT #
1	Hundred	1
2	Roll Up	2
3	Roll Over	54
4	Single Leg Circle	3
5	Single Leg Circle Full	30
6	Roll Like a Ball	4
7	Single Leg Pull Bent	5
8	Double Leg Pull Bent	6
9	Single Leg Pull Straight	9
10	Double Leg Straight	24
11	Criss Cross	25
12	Spine Stretch Forward	7
13	Open Leg Rocker	18
14	Corkscrew Flat	26
15	Corkscrew Tail Off	32
16	Corkscrew Full	49
17	Corkscrew Twist	63
18	Tick Tock	64
19	Saw	15
20	Neck Roll	27
21	Swan Preparation	38

The Order of Things
after Kneeling Side Kicks - Circles

PERFORMANCE ORDER	EXERCISE	ADD NEXT #
22	Single Leg Kick Back	14
23	Double Leg Kick Back	29
24	Thigh Stretch	59
25	The Neck Pull	31
26	Spine Twist	40
27	Jackknife	62
28	Side Kicks - Front & Back	21
29	Side Kicks - Up & Down	20
30	Side Kicks - Small Circles	22
31	Side Kicks - Medium Circles*	37
32	Side Kicks - Large Circles	48
33	Side Kicks - Inner Thigh Lifts*	42
34	Side Kicks - Inner Thigh Circles*	43
35	Side Kicks - Side Bicycle*	44
36	Side Kicks - Double Leg Lifts*	45
37	Side Kicks - Beats*	46
38	Side Kicks - Crosses*	47
39	Side Kicks - Bicycle	33
40	Side Kicks - Grand Circles *	53
41	Teaser 1	28
42	Teaser 2	41
43	Teaser 3	55
44	Hip Circles	56
45	Swimming	50
46	Leg Pull Front	57
47	Leg Pull Back	58
48	Kneeling Side Kicks - Front & Back	52
49	Kneeling Side Kicks - Up & Down	51
50	**KNEELING SIDE KICKS - CIRCLES**	**65**
51	Snake & Twist	61
52	Side Bend	60
53	Seal With Beats	34
54	Pilates Push Up	36

*optional if needed by student

Kneeling Side Kicks - Bicycle

Add Next	66
Pages	249-251
Thread(s)	Stability 34 Extension 17

Advanced:

- Baseline Variation: Goal Instructions
- Challenge Variation 1: Increase Range of Motion
  To challenge stability.
- Challenge Variation 2: Add Hold
  To challenge stability, stretch, and strength.

Super Advanced:

- Challenge Variation 3: Vigorous Pace
  To challenge Stability.
- Challenge Variation 4: Old Fashioned
  Teach before Star Old Fashioned on the Reformer.

The Order of Things
after Kneeling Side Kicks - Bicycles

PERFORMANCE ORDER	EXERCISE	ADD NEXT #
1	Hundred	1
2	Roll Up	2
3	Roll Over	54
4	Single Leg Circle	3
5	Single Leg Circle Full	30
6	Roll Like a Ball	4
7	Single Leg Pull Bent	5
8	Double Leg Pull Bent	6
9	Single Leg Pull Straight	9
10	Double Leg Straight	24
11	Criss Cross	25
12	Spine Stretch Forward	7
13	Open Leg Rocker	18
14	Corkscrew Flat	26
15	Corkscrew Tail Off	32
16	Corkscrew Full	49
17	Corkscrew Twist	63
18	Tick Tock	64
19	Saw	15
20	Neck Roll	27
21	Swan Preparation	38

The Order of Things
after Kneeling Side Kicks - Bicycles

PERFORMANCE ORDER	EXERCISE	ADD NEXT #
22	Single Leg Kick Back	14
23	Double Leg Kick Back	29
24	Thigh Stretch	59
25	The Neck Pull	31
26	Spine Twist	40
27	Jackknife	62
28	Side Kicks - Front & Back	21
29	Side Kicks - Up & Down	20
30	Side Kicks - Small Circles	22
31	Side Kicks - Medium Circles*	37
32	Side Kicks - Large Circles	48
33	Side Kicks - Inner Thigh Lifts*	42
34	Side Kicks - Inner Thigh Circles*	43
35	Side Kicks - Side Bicycle*	44
36	Side Kicks - Double Leg Lifts*	45
37	Side Kicks - Beats*	46
38	Side Kicks - Crosses*	47
39	Side Kicks - Bicycle	33
40	Side Kicks - Grand Circles *	53
41	Teaser 1	28
42	Teaser 2	41
43	Teaser 3	55
44	Hip Circles	56
45	Swimming	50
46	Leg Pull Front	57
47	Leg Pull Back	58
48	Kneeling Side Kicks - Front & Back	52
49	Kneeling Side Kicks - Up & Down	51
50	Kneeling Side Kicks - Circles	65
51	**KNEELING SIDE KICKS - BICYCLE**	**66**
52	Snake & Twist	61
53	Side Bend	60
54	Seal With Beats	34
55	Pilates Push Up	36

*optional, if needed by student

Rocking

Add Next	67
Pages	277-278
Thread(s)	Stability 35
	Extension 18
	Rolling (Extension) 5

Advanced:

- Building Variation 1: Single Leg Stretch
  For the student with one side tighter than the other.
- Baseline Variation: Goal Instructions

Super Advanced:

- Challenge Variation 2: Reverse Grip
  To open the shoulders as needed on the Rowing Series on the Reformer.

The Order of Things
after Rocking

PERFORMANCE ORDER	EXERCISE	ADD NEXT #
1	Hundred	1
2	Roll Up	2
3	Roll Over	54
4	Single Leg Circle	3
5	Single Leg Circle Full	30
6	Roll Like a Ball	4
7	Single Leg Pull Bent	5
8	Double Leg Pull Bent	6
9	Single Leg Pull Straight	9
10	Double Leg Straight	24
11	Criss Cross	25
12	Spine Stretch Forward	7
13	Open Leg Rocker	18
14	Corkscrew Flat	26
15	Corkscrew Tail Off	32
16	Corkscrew Full	49
17	Corkscrew Twist	63
18	Tick Tock	64
19	Saw	15
20	Neck Roll	27
21	Swan Preparation	38
22	Single Leg Kick Back	14
23	Double Leg Kick Back	29
24	Thigh Stretch	59
25	The Neck Pull	31
26	Spine Twist	40
27	Jackknife	62

The Order of Things
after Rocking

PERFORMANCE ORDER	EXERCISE	ADD NEXT #
28	Side Kicks - Front & Back	21
29	Side Kicks - Up & Down	20
30	Side Kicks - Small Circles	22
31	Side Kicks - Medium Circles*	37
32	Side Kicks - Large Circles	48
33	Side Kicks - Inner Thigh Lifts*	42
34	Side Kicks - Inner Thigh Circles*	43
35	Side Kicks - Side Bicycle*	44
36	Side Kicks - Double Leg Lifts*	45
37	Side Kicks - Beats*	46
38	Side Kicks - Crosses*	47
39	Side Kicks - Bicycle	33
40	Side Kicks - Grand Circles *	53
41	Teaser 1	28
42	Teaser 2	41
43	Teaser 3	55
44	Hip Circles	56
45	Swimming	50
46	Leg Pull Front	57
47	Leg Pull Back	58
48	Kneeling Side Kicks - Front & Back	52
49	Kneeling Side Kicks - Up & Down	51
50	Kneeling Side Kicks - Circles	65
51	Kneeling Side Kicks - Bicycle	66
52	Snake & Twist	61
53	Side Bend	60
54	Seal With Beats	34
55	**ROCKING**	**67**
56	Pilates Push Up	36

*optional, if needed by student

Swan Dive

Add Next	68
Pages	119-120
Thread(s)	Stability 36 Extension 19 Rolling (Extension) 6

Advanced:

- Baseline Variation: Goal Instructions

Super Advanced:

- Challenge Variation 1: Arms in Front
- Unofficial Challenge Variation (in Teaching section): Omit Hold

Note: When Swan Dive is added, Swan Preparation is omitted from the Performance Order.

The Order of Things
after Swan Dive

PERFORMANCE ORDER	EXERCISE	ADD NEXT #
1	Hundred	1
2	Roll Up	2
3	Roll Over	54
4	Single Leg Circle	3
5	Single Leg Circle Full	30
6	Roll Like a Ball	4
7	Single Leg Pull Bent	5
8	Double Leg Pull Bent	6
9	Single Leg Pull Straight	9
10	Double Leg Straight	24
11	Criss Cross	25
12	Spine Stretch Forward	7
13	Open Leg Rocker	18
14	Corkscrew Flat	26
15	Corkscrew Tail Off	32
16	Corkscrew Full	49
17	Corkscrew Twist	63
18	Tick Tock	64
19	Saw	15
20	Neck Roll	27
21	**SWAN DIVE**	**67**
22	Single Leg Kick Back	14
23	Double Leg Kick Back	29
24	Thigh Stretch	59
25	The Neck Pull	31
26	Spine Twist	40
27	Jackknife	62

The Order of Things
after Swan Dive

PERFORMANCE ORDER	EXERCISE	ADD NEXT #
28	Side Kicks - Front & Back	21
29	Side Kicks - Up & Down	20
30	Side Kicks - Small Circles	22
31	Side Kicks - Medium Circles*	37
32	Side Kicks - Large Circles	48
33	Side Kicks - Inner Thigh Lifts*	42
34	Side Kicks - Inner Thigh Circles*	43
35	Side Kicks - Side Bicycle*	44
36	Side Kicks - Double Leg Lifts*	45
37	Side Kicks - Beats*	46
38	Side Kicks - Crosses*	47
39	Side Kicks - Bicycle	33
40	Side Kicks - Grand Circles *	53
41	Teaser 1	28
42	Teaser 2	41
43	Teaser 3	55
44	Hip Circles	56
45	Swimming	50
46	Leg Pull Front	57
47	Leg Pull Back	58
48	Kneeling Side Kicks - Front & Back	52
49	Kneeling Side Kicks - Up & Down	51
50	Kneeling Side Kicks - Circles	65
51	Kneeling Side Kicks - Bicycle	66
52	Snake & Twist	61
53	Side Bend	60
54	Seal With Beats	34
55	Rocking	67
56	Pilates Push Up	36

*optional, if needed by student

Control Balance

Add Next	69
Pages	279-281
Thread(s)	Stability 37

Advanced:
- Building Variation 1: Two Legs Down
- Baseline Variation: Goal Instructions

Super Advanced:
- Challenge Variation 2: One Leg Stand
- Challenge Variation 3: Roll Back to Stand
  Use this variation to end the Control Balance Series and transition into the Push Up.

The Order of Things
after Control Balance

PERFORMANCE ORDER	EXERCISE	ADD NEXT #
1	Hundred	1
2	Roll Up	2
3	Roll Over	54
4	Single Leg Circle	3
5	Single Leg Circle Full	30
6	Roll Like a Ball	4
7	Single Leg Pull Bent	5
8	Double Leg Pull Bent	6
9	Single Leg Pull Straight	9
10	Double Leg Straight	24
11	Criss Cross	25
12	Spine Stretch Forward	7
13	Open Leg Rocker	18
14	Corkscrew Flat	26
15	Corkscrew Tail Off	32
16	Corkscrew Full	49
17	Corkscrew Twist	63
18	Tick Tock	64
19	Saw	15
20	Neck Roll	27
21	Swan Dive	67
22	Single Leg Kick Back	14
23	Double Leg Kick Back	29
24	Thigh Stretch	59
25	The Neck Pull	31
26	Spine Twist	40
27	Jackknife	62

The Order of Things
after Control Balance

PERFORMANCE ORDER	EXERCISE	ADD NEXT #
28	Side Kicks - Front & Back	21
29	Side Kicks - Up & Down	20
30	Side Kicks - Small Circles	22
31	Side Kicks - Medium Circles*	37
32	Side Kicks - Large Circles	48
33	Side Kicks - Inner Thigh Lifts*	42
34	Side Kicks - Inner Thigh Circles*	43
35	Side Kicks - Side Bicycle*	44
36	Side Kicks - Double Leg Lifts*	45
37	Side Kicks - Beats*	46
38	Side Kicks - Crosses*	47
39	Side Kicks - Bicycle	33
40	Side Kicks - Grand Circles *	53
41	Teaser 1	28
42	Teaser 2	41
43	Teaser 3	55
44	Hip Circles	56
45	Swimming	50
46	Leg Pull Front	57
47	Leg Pull Back	58
48	Kneeling Side Kicks - Front & Back	52
49	Kneeling Side Kicks - Up & Down	51
50	Kneeling Side Kicks - Circles	65
51	Kneeling Side Kicks - Bicycle	66
52	Snake & Twist	61
53	Side Bend	60
54	Seal With Beats	34
55	Rocking	67
56	**CONTROL BALANCE**	**69**
57	Pilates Push Up	36

*optional, if needed by student

Shoulder Bridge

Add Next	70
Pages	147-150
Thread(s)	Stability 38 Extension 20

Advanced:

- Unofficial Building Variation (in Teaching notes): Teach on Small Barrel or Spine Corrector
- Unofficial Building Variation (in Teaching notes): Flex & Point
  for tighter back of legs or to challenge coordination
- Baseline Variation: Goal Instructions

Super Advanced:

- Challenge Variation 1: Circles
  To challenge balance and stability.
- Challenge Variation 2: Bicycle
  To open the front of the hip and to prepare for the High Bridge (Add Next #77)
- Challenge Variation 3: Open Side
  To prepare for Balance Control Fan Kicks on the Reformer.
- Challenge Variation 4: Open Side/Lower & Lift Combo
  To prepare for Control Balance Fan Kicks on the Reformer.
- Challenge Variation 5: Fan
  To prepare for Control Balance Fan Kicks on the Reformer.
- Challenge Variation 6: Alternate Legs
  To prepare for Control Balance Fan Kicks on the Reformer

The Order of Things
after Shoulder Bridge

PERFORMANCE ORDER	EXERCISE	ADD NEXT #
1	Hundred	1
2	Roll Up	2
3	Roll Over	54
4	Single Leg Circle	3
5	Single Leg Circle Full	30
6	Roll Like a Ball	4
7	Single Leg Pull Bent	5
8	Double Leg Pull Bent	6
9	Single Leg Pull Straight	9
10	Double Leg Straight	24
11	Criss Cross	25
12	Spine Stretch Forward	7
13	Open Leg Rocker	18

The Order of Things
after Shoulder Bridge

PERFORMANCE ORDER	EXERCISE	ADD NEXT #
14	Corkscrew Flat	26
15	Corkscrew Tail Off	32
16	Corkscrew Full	49
17	Corkscrew Twist	63
18	Tick Tock	64
19	Saw	15
20	Neck Roll	27
21	Swan Dive	67
22	Single Leg Kick Back	14
23	Double Leg Kick Back	29
24	Thigh Stretch	59
25	The Neck Pull	31
26	**SHOULDER BRIDGE**	**70**
27	Spine Twist	40
28	Jackknife	62
29	Side Kicks - Front & Back	21
30	Side Kicks - Up & Down	20
31	Side Kicks - Small Circles	22
32	Side Kicks - Medium Circles*	37
33	Side Kicks - Large Circles	48
34	Side Kicks - Inner Thigh Lifts*	42
35	Side Kicks - Inner Thigh Circles*	43
36	Side Kicks - Side Bicycle*	44
37	Side Kicks - Double Leg Lifts*	45
38	Side Kicks - Beats*	46
39	Side Kicks - Crosses*	47
40	Side Kicks - Bicycle	33
41	Side Kicks - Grand Circles *	53
42	Teaser 1	28
43	Teaser 2	41
44	Teaser 3	55
45	Hip Circles	56
46	Swimming	50
47	Leg Pull Front	57
48	Leg Pull Back	58
49	Kneeling Side Kicks - Front & Back	52
50	Kneeling Side Kicks - Up & Down	51
51	Kneeling Side Kicks - Circles	65
52	Kneeling Side Kicks - Bicycle	66
53	Snake & Twist	61
54	Side Bend	60
55	Seal With Beats	34
56	Rocking	67
57	Control Balance	69
58	Pilates Push Up	36

*optional, if needed by student

Side Kicks -
Hot Potato

Advanced:

- Baseline Variation: Goal Instructions

Super Advanced:

- Challenge Variation 1: Idaho Potato
  In preparation for the Star Front and Back and the Tendon Stretch Combination on the Reformer.

The Order of Things
after Side Kick – Hot Potato

PERFORMANCE ORDER	EXERCISE	ADD NEXT #
1	Hundred	1
2	Roll Up	2
3	Roll Over	54
4	Single Leg Circle	3
5	Single Leg Circle Full	30
6	Roll Like a Ball	4
7	Single Leg Pull Bent	5
8	Double Leg Pull Bent	6
9	Single Leg Pull Straight	9
10	Double Leg Straight	24
11	Criss Cross	25
12	Spine Stretch Forward	7
13	Open Leg Rocker	18
14	Corkscrew Flat	26
15	Corkscrew Tail Off	32
16	Corkscrew Full	49
17	Corkscrew Twist	63
18	Tick Tock	64
19	Saw	15
20	Neck Roll	27
21	Swan Dive	67
22	Single Leg Kick Back	14
23	Double Leg Kick Back	29
24	Thigh Stretch	59
25	The Neck Pull	31
26	Shoulder Bridge	70
27	Spine Twist	40
28	Jackknife	62

The Order of Things
after Side Kick – Hot Potato

PERFORMANCE ORDER	EXERCISE	ADD NEXT #
29	Side Kicks - Front & Back	21
30	Side Kicks - Up & Down	20
31	Side Kicks - Small Circles	22
32	Side Kicks - Medium Circles*	37
33	Side Kicks - Large Circles	48
34	Side Kicks - Inner Thigh Lifts*	42
35	Side Kicks - Inner Thigh Circles*	43
36	Side Kicks - Side Bicycle*	44
37	Side Kicks - Double Leg Lifts*	45
38	Side Kicks - Beats*	46
39	Side Kicks - Crosses*	47
40	Side Kicks - Bicycle	33
41	Side Kicks - Grand Circles *	53
42	**SIDE KICKS - HOT POTATO***	**71**
43	Teaser 1	28
44	Teaser 2	41
45	Teaser 3	55
46	Hip Circles	56
47	Swimming	50
48	Leg Pull Front	57
49	Leg Pull Back	58
50	Kneeling Side Kicks - Front & Back	52
51	Kneeling Side Kicks - Up & Down	51
52	Kneeling Side Kicks - Circles	65
53	Kneeling Side Kicks - Bicycle	66
54	Snake & Twist	61
55	Side Bend	60
56	Seal With Beats	34
57	Rocking	67
58	Control Balance	69
59	Pilates Push Up	36

*optional, if needed by student

Side Kicks -
Big Scissors

Add Next	72
Pages	199-200
Thread(s)	Stability 40 Extension 21

Advanced:

- Baseline Variation: Goal Instructions

Super Advanced:

- Challenge Variation 1: Double Bicycle
  To challenge stability during dynamic action and functional movement.

The Order of Things
after Side Kick – Big Scissors

PERFORMANCE ORDER	EXERCISE	ADD NEXT #
1	Hundred	1
2	Roll Up	2
3	Roll Over	54
4	Single Leg Circle	3
5	Single Leg Circle Full	30
6	Roll Like a Ball	4
7	Single Leg Pull Bent	5
8	Double Leg Pull Bent	6
9	Single Leg Pull Straight	9
10	Double Leg Straight	24
11	Criss Cross	25
12	Spine Stretch Forward	7
13	Open Leg Rocker	18
14	Corkscrew Flat	26
15	Corkscrew Tail Off	32
16	Corkscrew Full	49
17	Corkscrew Twist	63
18	Tick Tock	64
19	Saw	15
20	Neck Roll	27
21	Swan Dive	67
22	Single Leg Kick Back	14
23	Double Leg Kick Back	29
24	Thigh Stretch	59
25	The Neck Pull	31
26	Shoulder Bridge	70
27	Spine Twist	40
28	Jackknife	62

The Order of Things
after Side Kick – Big Scissors

PERFORMANCE ORDER	EXERCISE	ADD NEXT #
29	Side Kicks - Front & Back	21
30	Side Kicks - Up & Down	20
31	Side Kicks - Small Circles	22
32	Side Kicks - Medium Circles*	37
33	Side Kicks - Large Circles	48
34	Side Kicks - Inner Thigh Lifts*	42
35	Side Kicks - Inner Thigh Circles*	43
36	Side Kicks - Side Bicycle*	44
37	Side Kicks - Double Leg Lifts*	45
38	Side Kicks - Beats*	46
39	Side Kicks - Crosses*	47
40	Side Kicks - Bicycle	33
41	Side Kicks - Grand Circles *	53
42	Side Kicks - Hot Potato*	71
43	**SIDE KICKS - BIG SCISSORS***	**72**
44	Teaser 1	28
45	Teaser 2	41
46	Teaser 3	55
47	Hip Circles	56
48	Swimming	50
49	Leg Pull Front	57
50	Leg Pull Back	58
51	Kneeling Side Kicks - Front & Back	52
52	Kneeling Side Kicks - Up & Down	51
53	Kneeling Side Kicks - Circles	65
54	Kneeling Side Kicks - Bicycle	66
55	Snake & Twist	61
56	Side Bend	60
57	Seal With Beats	34
58	Rocking	67
59	Control Balance	69
60	Pilates Push Up	36

*optional, if needed by student

Boomerang

Add Next	73
Pages	265-269
Thread(s)	Rolling (Forward) 6

Advanced:

- Baseline Variation: Goal Instructions

Super Advanced:

- Challenge Variation 1: Teaser
  For increased control.
- Challenge Variation 2: Teaser Arms Front
  For increased control.
- Challenge Variation 3: Rolling Boomerang
  For dynamic action and to prepare for complete rolls in Roll Like a Ball (Roll Like a Ball, Add Next #4, Challenge Variations 9-13)
- Challenge Variation 4: Open Chest

The Order of Things
after Boomerang

PERFORMANCE ORDER	EXERCISE	ADD NEXT #
1	Hundred	1
2	Roll Up	2
3	Roll Over	54
4	Single Leg Circle	3
5	Single Leg Circle Full	30
6	Roll Like a Ball	4
7	Single Leg Pull Bent	5
8	Double Leg Pull Bent	6
9	Single Leg Pull Straight	9
10	Double Leg Straight	24
11	Criss Cross	25
12	Spine Stretch Forward	7
13	Open Leg Rocker	18
14	Corkscrew Flat	26
15	Corkscrew Tail Off	32
16	Corkscrew Full	49
17	Corkscrew Twist	63
18	Tick Tock	64
19	Saw	15
20	Neck Roll	27
21	Swan Dive	67
22	Single Leg Kick Back	14
23	Double Leg Kick Back	29

The Order of Things
after Boomerang

PERFORMANCE ORDER	EXERCISE	ADD NEXT #
24	Thigh Stretch	59
25	The Neck Pull	31
26	Shoulder Bridge	70
27	Spine Twist	40
28	Jackknife	62
29	Side Kicks - Front & Back	21
30	Side Kicks - Up & Down	20
31	Side Kicks - Small Circles	22
32	Side Kicks - Medium Circles*	37
33	Side Kicks - Large Circles	48
34	Side Kicks - Inner Thigh Lifts*	42
35	Side Kicks - Inner Thigh Circles*	43
36	Side Kicks - Side Bicycle*	44
37	Side Kicks - Double Leg Lifts*	45
38	Side Kicks - Beats*	46
39	Side Kicks - Crosses*	47
40	Side Kicks - Bicycle	33
41	Side Kicks - Grand Circles *	53
42	Side Kicks - Hot Potato*	71
43	Side Kicks - Big Scissors*	72
44	Teaser 1	28
45	Teaser 2	41
46	Teaser 3	55
47	Hip Circles	56
48	Swimming	50
49	Leg Pull Front	57
50	Leg Pull Back	58
51	Kneeling Side Kicks - Front & Back	52
52	Kneeling Side Kicks - Up & Down	51
53	Kneeling Side Kicks - Circles	65
54	Kneeling Side Kicks - Bicycle	66
55	Snake & Twist	61
56	Side Bend	60
57	**BOOMERANG**	**73**
58	Seal With Beats	34
59	Rocking	67
60	Control Balance	69
61	Pilates Push Up	36

*optional, if needed by student

High Scissors

Add Next	74
Pages	141-142
Thread(s)	Stability 41 Extension 22

Advanced:

- Baseline Variation: Goal Instructions

Super Advanced:

- Challenge Variation 1: Toe Touch
  To prepare for High Bridge One Leg.
- Challenge Variation 2: Scissors Overhead
  To stretch the back body to prepare for Control Balance One Leg to Stand (Add Next #69, Challenge Variation 2).
- Challenge Variation 3: Split Scissors
  Prepares for Split Walks and Control Balance Off on the Reformer.

The Order of Things
after High Scissors

PERFORMANCE ORDER	EXERCISE	ADD NEXT #
1	Hundred	1
2	Roll Up	2
3	Roll Over	54
4	Single Leg Circle	3
5	Single Leg Circle Full	30
6	Roll Like a Ball	4
7	Single Leg Pull Bent	5
8	Double Leg Pull Bent	6
9	Single Leg Pull Straight	9
10	Double Leg Straight	24
11	Criss Cross	25
12	Spine Stretch Forward	7
13	Open Leg Rocker	18
14	Corkscrew Flat	26
15	Corkscrew Tail Off	32
16	Corkscrew Full	49
17	Corkscrew Twist	63
18	Tick Tock	64
19	Saw	15
20	Neck Roll	27
21	Swan Dive	67
22	Single Leg Kick Back	14
23	Double Leg Kick Back	29

The Order of Things
after High Scissors

PERFORMANCE ORDER	EXERCISE	ADD NEXT #
24	Thigh Stretch	59
25	The Neck Pull	31
26	**HIGH SCISSORS**	**74**
27	Shoulder Bridge	70
28	Spine Twist	40
29	Jackknife	62
30	Side Kicks - Front & Back	21
31	Side Kicks - Up & Down	20
32	Side Kicks - Small Circles	22
33	Side Kicks - Medium Circles*	37
34	Side Kicks - Large Circles	48
35	Side Kicks - Inner Thigh Lifts*	42
36	Side Kicks - Inner Thigh Circles*	43
37	Side Kicks - Side Bicycle*	44
38	Side Kicks - Double Leg Lifts*	45
39	Side Kicks - Beats*	46
40	Side Kicks - Crosses*	47
41	Side Kicks - Bicycle	33
42	Side Kicks - Grand Circles *	53
43	Side Kicks - Hot Potato*	71
44	Side Kicks - Big Scissors*	72
45	Teaser 1	28
46	Teaser 2	41
47	Teaser 3	55
48	Hip Circles	56
49	Swimming	50
50	Leg Pull Front	57
51	Leg Pull Back	58
52	Kneeling Side Kicks - Front & Back	52
53	Kneeling Side Kicks - Up & Down	51
54	Kneeling Side Kicks - Circles	65
55	Kneeling Side Kicks - Bicycle	66
56	Snake & Twist	61
57	Side Bend	60
58	Boomerang	73
59	Seal With Beats	34
60	Rocking	67
61	Control Balance	69
62	Pilates Push Up	36

*optional, if needed by student

High Bicycle

Add Next	75
Pages	143-145
Thread(s)	Stability 42 Extension 23

Advanced:

- Baseline Variation: Goal Instructions

Super Advanced:

- Challenge Variation 1: Toe Touch
  Open the front of the hip; prepares for High Bridge One Leg (Add Next #77, Challenge Variations 2-4 and 6)
- Challenge Variation 2: Bicycle Overhead
  Stretches back body; prepares for Control Balance One Leg to Stand (Add Next #69, Challenge Variation 2)
- Challenge Variation 3: Split Bicycle Scissors
  Prepares for Split Walks and Control Balance Off on the Reformer.

PERFORMANCE ORDER	EXERCISE	ADD NEXT #
1	Hundred	1
2	Roll Up	2
3	Roll Over	54
4	Single Leg Circle	3
5	Single Leg Circle Full	30
6	Roll Like a Ball	4
7	Single Leg Pull Bent	5
8	Double Leg Pull Bent	6
9	Single Leg Pull Straight	9
10	Double Leg Straight	24
11	Criss Cross	25
12	Spine Stretch Forward	7
13	Open Leg Rocker	18
14	Corkscrew Flat	26
15	Corkscrew Tail Off	32
16	Corkscrew Full	49
17	Corkscrew Twist	63
18	Tick Tock	64
19	Saw	15
20	Neck Roll	27
21	Swan Dive	67
22	Single Leg Kick Back	14
23	Double Leg Kick Back	29

The Order of Things
after High Bicycle

PERFORMANCE ORDER	EXERCISE	ADD NEXT #
24	Thigh Stretch	59
25	The Neck Pull	31
26	High Scissors	74
27	**HIGH BICYCLE**	**75**
28	Shoulder Bridge	70
29	Spine Twist	40
30	Jackknife	62
31	Side Kicks - Front & Back	21
32	Side Kicks - Up & Down	20
33	Side Kicks - Small Circles	22
34	Side Kicks - Medium Circles*	37
35	Side Kicks - Large Circles	48
36	Side Kicks - Inner Thigh Lifts*	42
37	Side Kicks - Inner Thigh Circles*	43
38	Side Kicks - Side Bicycle*	44
39	Side Kicks - Double Leg Lifts*	45
40	Side Kicks - Beats*	46
41	Side Kicks - Crosses*	47
42	Side Kicks - Bicycle	33
43	Side Kicks - Grand Circles *	53
44	Side Kicks - Hot Potato*	71
45	Side Kicks - Big Scissors*	72
46	Teaser 1	28
47	Teaser 2	41
48	Teaser 3	55
49	Hip Circles	56
50	Swimming	50
51	Leg Pull Front	57
52	Leg Pull Back	58
53	Kneeling Side Kicks - Front & Back	52
54	Kneeling Side Kicks - Up & Down	51
55	Kneeling Side Kicks - Circles	65
56	Kneeling Side Kicks - Bicycle	66
57	Snake & Twist	61
58	Side Bend	60
59	Boomerang	73
60	Seal With Beats	34
61	Rocking	67
62	Control Balance	69
63	Pilates Push Up	36

*optional, if needed by student

Crab

Add Next	76
Pages	275-276
Thread(s)	Rolling (Forward) 7

Advanced:

- Baseline Variation: Goal Instructions

Super Advanced:

- Challenge Variation 1: Lifted Feet

The Order of Things
after Crab

PERFORMANCE ORDER	EXERCISE	ADD NEXT #
1	Hundred	1
2	Roll Up	2
3	Roll Over	54
4	Single Leg Circle	3
5	Single Leg Circle Full	30
6	Roll Like a Ball	4
7	Single Leg Pull Bent	5
8	Double Leg Pull Bent	6
9	Single Leg Pull Straight	9
10	Double Leg Straight	24
11	Criss Cross	25
12	Spine Stretch Forward	7
13	Open Leg Rocker	18
14	Corkscrew Flat	26
15	Corkscrew Tail Off	32
16	Corkscrew Full	49
17	Corkscrew Twist	63
18	Tick Tock	64
19	Saw	15
20	Neck Roll	27
21	Swan Dive	67
22	Single Leg Kick Back	14
23	Double Leg Kick Back	29
24	Thigh Stretch	59
25	The Neck Pull	31
26	High Scissors	74
27	High Bicycle	75
28	Shoulder Bridge	70
29	Spine Twist	40
30	Jackknife	62

The Order of Things
after Crab

PERFORMANCE ORDER	EXERCISE	ADD NEXT #
31	Side Kicks - Front & Back	21
32	Side Kicks - Up & Down	20
33	Side Kicks - Small Circles	22
34	Side Kicks - Medium Circles*	37
35	Side Kicks - Large Circles	48
36	Side Kicks - Inner Thigh Lifts*	42
37	Side Kicks - Inner Thigh Circles*	43
38	Side Kicks - Side Bicycle*	44
39	Side Kicks - Double Leg Lifts*	45
40	Side Kicks - Beats*	46
41	Side Kicks - Crosses*	47
42	Side Kicks - Bicycle	33
43	Side Kicks - Grand Circles *	53
44	Side Kicks - Hot Potato*	71
45	Side Kicks - Big Scissors*	72
46	Teaser 1	28
47	Teaser 2	41
48	Teaser 3	55
49	Hip Circles	56
50	Swimming	50
51	Leg Pull Front	57
52	Leg Pull Back	58
53	Kneeling Side Kicks - Front & Back	52
54	Kneeling Side Kicks - Up & Down	51
55	Kneeling Side Kicks - Circles	65
56	Kneeling Side Kicks - Bicycle	66
57	Snake & Twist	61
58	Side Bend	60
59	Boomerang	73
60	Seal With Beats	34
61	**CRAB**	**76**
62	Rocking	67
63	Control Balance	69
64	Pilates Push Up	36

*optional, if needed by student

High Bridge

Add Next	77
Pages	291-293
Thread(s)	Stability 43 Extension 22

Advanced 2:

- Building Variation 1: Use Handles
- Baseline Variation: Goal Instructions

Super Advanced:

- Challenge Variation 2: Single Leg Bend/Extend
  Prepares for High Bridge on the Reformer.
- Challenge Variation 3: Single Leg Slide & Lift
  Prepares for High Bridge on the Reformer.
- Challenge Variation 4: Single Leg Bend/Extend/Slide Combo (Bicycle)
  Prepares for High Bridge on the Reformer.
- Challenge Variation 5: Single Arm
  Challenges upper body stretch, strength & control.
- Challenge Variation 6: Single Arm & Single Leg
  To challenge balance, stretch, strength & control.

The Order of Things
after High Bridge

PERFORMANCE ORDER	EXERCISE	ADD NEXT #
1	Hundred	1
2	Roll Up	2
3	Roll Over	54
4	Single Leg Circle	3
5	Single Leg Circle Full	30
6	Roll Like a Ball	4
7	Single Leg Pull Bent	5
8	Double Leg Pull Bent	6
9	Single Leg Pull Straight	9
10	Double Leg Straight	24
11	Criss Cross	25
12	Spine Stretch Forward	7
13	Open Leg Rocker	18
14	Corkscrew Flat	26
15	Corkscrew Tail Off	32
16	Corkscrew Full	49
17	Corkscrew Twist	63
18	Tick Tock	64
19	Saw	15
20	Neck Roll	27
21	Swan Dive	67
22	Single Leg Kick Back	14
23	Double Leg Kick Back	29

The Order of Things
after High Bridge

PERFORMANCE ORDER	EXERCISE	ADD NEXT #
24	Thigh Stretch	59
25	The Neck Pull	31
26	High Scissors	74
27	High Bicycle	75
28	Shoulder Bridge	70
29	Spine Twist	40
30	Jackknife	62
31	Side Kicks - Front & Back	21
32	Side Kicks - Up & Down	20
33	Side Kicks - Small Circles	22
34	Side Kicks - Medium Circles*	37
35	Side Kicks - Large Circles	48
36	Side Kicks - Inner Thigh Lifts*	42
37	Side Kicks - Inner Thigh Circles*	43
38	Side Kicks - Side Bicycle*	44
39	Side Kicks - Double Leg Lifts*	45
40	Side Kicks - Beats*	46
41	Side Kicks - Crosses*	47
42	Side Kicks - Bicycle	33
43	Side Kicks - Grand Circles *	53
44	Side Kicks - Hot Potato*	71
45	Side Kicks - Big Scissors*	72
46	Teaser 1	28
47	Teaser 2	41
48	Teaser 3	55
49	Hip Circles	56
50	Swimming	50
51	Leg Pull Front	57
52	Leg Pull Back	58
53	Kneeling Side Kicks - Front & Back	52
54	Kneeling Side Kicks - Up & Down	51
55	Kneeling Side Kicks - Circles	65
56	Kneeling Side Kicks - Bicycle	66
57	Snake & Twist	61
58	Side Bend	60
59	Boomerang	73
60	Seal With Beats	34
61	Crab	76
62	Rocking	67
63	Control Balance	69
64	Pilates Push Up	36
65	**HIGH BRIDGE**	**77**

*optional, if needed by student

5. PROGRESSION CHECKLIST

There are likely to be variations your body isn't ready for, even in the early exercises. Use the chart below to track which variations you've explored and which ones you need to come back to. Both the page number for *The Red Thread*© (RT PAGE) and the page of this Study Guide (SG PAGE) are listed. Variations in [brackets] are not noted as Variations in *The Red Thread*© but are found somewhere in the text.

ADD NEXT	EXERCISE NAME	RT PAGE	SG PAGE
	LEVEL VARIATION TYPE: NAME		
1	**Hundred**	29	22
	F BV 1: Legs Flat on the Mat		
	F BV 2: Barrel		
	C BV 3: Single Leg Lift & Lower		
	C BV 4: Single Leg Lower & Lift		
	C BV 5: Double Leg Lower & Lift		
	C BV 6: Parallel Lines		
	C Baseline – Goal Instructions		
	A CV 7: Heel Beats		
	A CV 8: Walking		
	A CV 9: Weighted Bar		
2	**Roll Up**	35	23
	F BV 1: Roll Up - Hand Slide		
	F BV 2: Roll Back		
	F BV 3: Roll Down		
	F BV 4: Speed Bump		
	F BV 5: Teacher Holds Bar		
	C BV 6: Hook the Foot		
	C BV 7: Hand Slide on Full Roll Up		
	C Baseline – Goal		
	A CV 8: Roll Up with Pointed Feet		
	A CV 9: Pause		
	A CV 10: Up Two – Down One		
	A CV 11: Wide Grip		
3	**Single Leg Circle**	45	24
	F BV 1: Bent Knee – Sign of the Cross		
	F BV 2: Bent Knee – Small Circles		
	F BV 3: Small Circles with Bent Base Knee		
	F BV 4: Small Circles with Wide Base		
	F Baseline – Goal Instructions through step 10		
	SA CV 5: Arm Overhead with Weights		
	SA CV 6: Lifted Bottom Leg		

CHART LEGEND

Levels
F   Foundational
F2 Foundational 2
C   Core
A   Advanced
SA Super Advanced

Variation Types
BV   Building Variation
CV   Challenge Variation
[BV] Unofficial Building Variation
[CV] Unofficial Challenge Variation

4		**Roll Like a Ball**	55	25
	F	BV 1: Roll Back		
	F	Baseline – Goal Instructions		
	C	CV 2: Full Roll to Shoulders		
	C	CV 3: Accent		
	A	CV 4: Advanced Hand Position		
	A	CV 5: Hold and Balance		
	A	CV 6: Shoulder Stand into Roll		
	A	CV 7: Teaser into Roll		
	A	CV 8: Teaser Shoulder Stand Combo		
	A	CV 9: Roll to Stand		
	A	CV 10: Roll to Jump		
	A	CV 11: Stand with Single Leg Front		
	A	CV 12: Stand with Single Leg Front into Kneeling Knee Scale on Foot into Backbend		
	A	CV 13: Single Leg Russian Roll		
	A	CV 14: Elbows to Knees		
5		**Single Leg Pull Bent**	59	27
	F	BV 1: Change with Two Legs into Chest		
	F	BV 2: Fluid Change		
	F	Baseline: Goal Instructions		
	C	CV 3: Teaser Change		
	A	CV 4: Extended Leg Pause		
	A	CV 5: Slice Off Bottom (Bicycle)		
	A	CV 6: No Hands		
	SA	CV 7: Rolling Up into Teaser		
6		**Double Leg Pull Bent**	63	28
	F	BV 1: Arms by Sides		
	F	BV 2: Hand Slide on Legs		
	C	BV 3: Arms Straight Back & In		
	C	BV 4: No Hands		
	C	Baseline: Goal Instructions		
	A	CV 5: Back Stroke		
	A	CV 6: Count Hold Arm Circles		
	A	CV 7: Fully Open		
	A	CV 8: Backstroke Swimming		
	A	CV 9: Around the Clock		

27	**Neck Roll**		113	55
	C	Baseline: Goal Instructions		
28	**Teaser 1**		215	56
	C	Baseline: Goal Instructions		
	A	CV 1: Seated Teaser		
	A	CV 2: Half Way Down		
	SA	CV 3: Arms to Ears		
29	**Double Leg Kick Back**		125	58
	C	BV 1: Single Leg Stretch		
	C	Baseline: Goal Instructions		
	C	CV 2: Clasped Hands on Buttocks		
	C	CV 3: Clasped Hands Lifted		
	C	CV 4: Flat Hands Palms Face Up		
	C	CV 5: Finger Tip Elbow		
	C	CV 6: Reverse Prayer Palms Up		
	SA	CV 7: Lift Legs Off Mat		
30	**Single Leg Circle Full**		53	60
	C	Baseline: Goal Instructions		
	SA	CV 1: Lift Bottom Leg		
31	**The Neck Pull**		135	62
	C	BV 1: Two Up One Down		
	C	BV 2: Elbows In		
	C	BV 3: Pause		
	C	BV 4: No Pulse		
	C	Baseline: Goal Instructions		
	A	CV 5: Flat Back		
32	**Corkscrew Tail Off**		101	64
	C	BV 1: Sign of the Cross – Hip Lift		
	C	Baseline: Goal Instructions		
33	**Side Kicks - Bicycle**		189	65
	C	Baseline: Goal Instructions		
	A	CV 1: Pause		
	SA	CV 2: Hold & Stretch		
34	**Seal With Beats**		273	66
	C	Baseline: Goal Instructions		
	A	CV 1: Inch Balance		
	A	CV 2: Extended Seal		
35	**Can Can**		227	67
	C	BV 1: Simple Can Can		
	C	BV 2: Can Can Elbows to Mat		
	C	Baseline: Goal Instructions		
	C	CV 3: Reverse Can Can		

40	**Spine Twist**		151	76
	C2	[BV]: Feet pressed against a wall		
	C2	BV 1: Hands on Shoulders		
	C2	BV 2: Clasped Hands – Flat Hands		
	C2	BV 3: Fingertip to Elbow		
	C2	BV 4: Hand to Shoulder – Elbows Down		
	C2	Baseline: Goal Instructions		
	A	CV 5: Prayer Hands		
	A	CV 6: One Arm Up – One Arm Down		
	A	CV 7: Pole Looped Over		
	A	CV 8: Pole Looped Under – Ribs On & Ribs Off		
	SA	CV 9: Pulse		
	SA	CV 10: Head Turn		
	SA	CV 11: Wide Arms		
	SA	CV 12: Reversed Breathing		
41	**Teaser 2**		219	78
	C2	Baseline: Goal Instructions		
	A	CV 1: Arms to Ears		
	SA	CV 2: Circles in Opposition		
42	**Side Kicks - Inner Thigh Lifts**		175	80
	C	BV 1: Increase Repetitions		
	C	BV 2: Quick Lower & Lift		
	C	Baseline: Goal Instructions		
	A	CV 3: Increase Dynamics		
	SA	CV 4: Add Hold on Lift		
43	**Side Kicks - Inner Thigh Circle**		177	82
	C2	BV 1: Increase Repetitions		
	C2	BV 2: Quick Circles		
	C2	Baseline: Goal Instructions		
	A	CV 3: Increase Dynamics		
	SA	CV 4: Add Hold on Lift		
44	**Side Kicks - Side Bicycle**		179	84
	C2	Baseline: Goal Instructions		
	A	CV 1: Both Hands Behind the Head		
	SA	CV 2: Hold & Stretch		
45	**Side Kicks - Double Leg Lifts**		183	86
	C2	Baseline: Goal Instructions		
	A	CV 1: Upper Body Lift		
	SA	CV 2: Fish		
46	**Side Kicks - Beats**		185	88
	C2	Baseline: Goal Instructions		
	A	CV 1: Increase Repetitions		
	SA	CV 2: Large Beats		
	SA	CV 3: Alternating Accent		

55		**Teaser 3**	221	106
	A	BV 1: Arms by Side		
	A	Baseline: Goal Instructions		
	A	CV 2: Arms to Ceiling Roll Back		
	A	CV 3: Arms to Ceiling Reach Back		
	A	CV 4: Arm by Ears		
	SA	CV 5: Toe Touches		
	SA	CV 6: Open Circle Legs & Arms in Opposition		
	SA	CV 7: Twisting		
	SA	CV 8: Walking		
	SA	CV 9: Beat Legs		
	SA	CV 10: Close Envelope – Open Envelope		
	SA	CV 11: Twisting 2		
	SA	CV 12: Pelvic Stability		
	SA	CV 13: Rowing Series		
	SA	CV 14: Shaving		
	SA	CV 15: Swan Dive Teaser Combination		
56		**Hip Circles**	229	108
	A	BV 1: Bent Arms Mat		
	A	BV 2: Bent Elbows		
	A	BV 3: Lifted Single Leg Tick Tock 1		
	A	BV 4: Lifted Single Leg Tick Tock 2		
	A	BV 5: Windshield Wiper		
	A	Baseline: Goal Instructions		
	SA	CV 6: Teacher's Stretch		
	SA	CV 7: Leg Toss Side to Side		
	SA	CV 8: Touch & Pause		
	SA	CV 9: Sweep		
57		**Leg Pull Front**	237	110
	A	[BV]: No Pulse		
	A	Baseline: Goal Instructions		
	SA	CV 1: Leg High		
	SA	CV 2: Leg Side		
	SA	CV 3: Leg Back & Side Combo		
	SA	CV 4: Lifted Arm		
58		**Leg Pull Back**	239	112
	A	Baseline: Goal Instructions		
	A	[CV]: Point Up, Flex Down		
	A	[CV]: Flexed Feet		
	SA	CV 1: Leg Side		
	SA	CV 2: Leg Side & Up		

	A	CV 2: Add Accent		
	A	CV 3: Vigorous Pace		
	SA	CV 4: Hold		
66		**Kneeling Side Kicks - Bicycle**	**249**	**128**
	A	Baseline: Goal Instructions		
	A	CV 1: Increase Range of Motion		
	A	CV 2: Add Hold		
	SA	CV 3: Vigorous Pace		
	SA	CV 4: Old Fashioned		
67		**Rocking**	**277**	**130**
	A	BV 1: Single Leg Stretch		
	A	Baseline: Goal Instructions		
	SA	CV 2: Reverse Grip		
68		**Swan Dive**	**119**	**132**
	A	Baseline: Goal Instructions		
	SA	CV 1: Arms in Front		
	SA	[CV]: Omit Hold		
69		**Control Balance**	**279**	**134**
	A	BV 1: Two Legs Down		
	A	Baseline: Goal Instructions		
	SA	CV 2: One Leg Stand		
	SA	CV 3: Roll Back to Stand		
70		**Shoulder Bridge**	**147**	**136**
	A	[BV]: Small Barrel or Spine Corrector		
	A	[BV]: Flex & Point		
	A	Baseline: Goal Instructions		
	SA	CV 1: Circles		
	SA	CV 2: Bicycle		
	SA	CV 3: Open Side		
	SA	CV 4: Open Side/Lower & Lift Combo		
	SA	CV 5: Fan		
	SA	CV 6: Alternate Legs		
71		**Side Kicks - Hot Potato**	**197**	**138**
	A	Baseline: Goal Instructions		
	SA	CV 1: Idaho Potato		
72		**Side Kicks - Big Scissors**	**199**	**140**
	A	Baseline: Goal Instructions		
	SA	CV 1: Double Bicycle		
73		**Boomerang**	**265**	**142**
	A	Baseline: Goal Instructions		
	SA	CV 1: Teaser		
	SA	CV 2: Teaser Arms Front		
	SA	CV 3: Rolling Boomerang		
	SA	CV 4: Open Chest		

6. FINAL THOUGHTS

Pilates, for me, is about connections. Our bodies are not disconnected parts - we are a beautifully connected whole. Kathi's book shows the beautiful connections of the Pilates Mat repertoire - not disconnected parts assembled willy-nilly but one flowing, continuous, *connected* series of related movements, each logically connected to each other.

I hope this Study Guide helps you see the connections Kathi has laid out for us, discover some of your own, and that this new vision of The Pilates Method inspires you to be thoughtful in building your mat workout routines.

7. ABOUT THE AUTHOR

Tracy Maurstad is an integrated health practitioner drawing from a wide range of study, certifications and experience. Her numerous areas of expertise include flexibility, strength, movement, fascia, nutrition, psychology, Pilates and the Nia Technique. Tracy is a lifelong student of healthy and natural living. Her wide range of study and more than 30 years of experience give her a uniquely informed point of view on living life with spontaneous Zest and Pleasure.

Tracy maintains a small private practice. She also organizes teacher trainings and publishes in the hope of helping many others achieve a healthy, happy and well-balanced life.

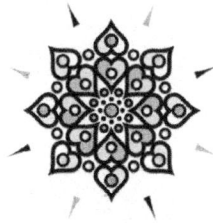

zest and pleasure
ZESTANDPLEASURE.COM

INDEX

Made in the USA
Las Vegas, NV
30 April 2023